Pulse Oximetry

Second edition

Pulse Oximetry

Second edition

John TB Moyle

*Chartered Engineer, Consultant in Palliative Medicine,
Milton Keynes General Hospital, and Medical Director,
Willen Hospice, Milton Keynes*

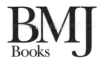

© BMJ Books 2002
BMJ Books is an imprint of the BMJ Publishing Group

First published in 1994
by BMJ Books, BMA House, Tavistock Square,
London WC1H 9JR

First edition 1994
Revised edition 1998
Second edition 2002

www.bmjbooks.com

British Library Cataloguing in Publication Data

A catalogue record for this book is available from the British Library

ISBN 0 7279 1740 4

Typeset by SIVA Math Setters, Chennai, India
Printed and bound in Spain by GraphyCems, Navarra

Contents

Acknowledgements

Certain authors, when they speak of their work, say "my book", "my comments", "my history".... They would be better to say "... our book", "our commentary", "our history", since their writings generally contain more of other people's good things than their own.

Blaise Pascal (1623–62)

For the Lord gives wisdom and from his mouth come knowledge and understanding.

Proverbs 2:6

I would like to thank the staff at Library of Postgraduate Centre, Milton Keynes General Hospital, for their help. I would also like to thank Professor W G Zijlstra of the Department of Physiology, University of Groningen, The Netherlands, for providing the data on which the absorption spectra in this book are based.

Introduction

The unreliability of cyanosis in the recognition of arterial hypoxaemia was highlighted in a classic paper by Comroe and Botelho,[1] who showed that 11% of a group of experienced clinicians could not detect cyanosis when the arterial oxygen saturation in healthy individuals had been reduced to 75%. Lundsgaard and Van Slyke[2] summarised the factors that contribute to the presence of cyanosis, and concluded that approximately 5 g reduced haemoglobin per 100 ml capillary blood must be present to produce visible cyanosis. The detection of cyanosis depends on variables in the patient, the environment and the observer. It is a poor guide to the detection of arterial hypoxaemia. Under the very best conditions desaturation is unlikely to be noticed clinically until it has fallen below 85%.

Before the development of pulse oximetry, numerous attempts at instrumentation for the detection of hypoxaemia were made; these are discussed in Chapter 1. These devices were unable to separate the arterial oxygen saturation from that of the venous and capillary blood, and it was not until the era of microprocessor technology that this separation could be made.

Pulse oximetry, which can differentiate between arterial blood (which is pulsatile) and venous capillary blood (which is smooth flowing), has in 15 years changed from a new monitoring technique to one which in some countries is mandatory with every general anaesthetic. It must surely be the ultimate safety monitor for use during anaesthesia, as it shows not only how well the patient is oxygenated, but also that the blood is circulating. It has the advantages of being non-invasive and of apparently having no morbidity, negligible running costs and a comparatively low capital cost. However, as with most new technologies, lack of knowledge of its underlying principles and limitations can lead to unjust criticism. Suprisingly for such a non-invasive technique, there have recently been reports of *morbidity* from pulse oximetry, in the form of tissue damage adjacent to the probe, and this has even led to a Safety Action Bulletin being issued by the Medical Devices Agency in England.[3]

This book gives a historical background, followed by a description of how pulse oximetry works. The problems of calibration are discussed, including a description of the "gold standard" against which pulse oximeters are calibrated – namely, the CO-oximeter. The clinical uses of pulse oximetry are characterised, and the limitations of the technique classified and described in detail.

Apart from general updating, this edition also deals with pulse oximetry at high altitude and when flying in aircraft, and there is a chapter on fetal pulse oximetry which was introduced in the revised reprint of the first edition.

1 Comroe JH, Botelho S. The unreliability of cyanosis in the recognition of arterial anoxemia. *Am J Med Sci* 1947;**214**:1–6.
2 Lundsgaard C, Van Slyke DD. Cyanosis. *Medicine* 1923;2:1.
3 Tissue necrosis caused by pulse oximeter probes. MDA SN2001(08) Medical Devices Agency, UK.

1: History of oxygen saturation monitoring

The relationship between the absorption of light and the amount of absorbant was first described by Johann Heinrich Lambert (1728–77) in Augsberg, Germany, and published by him in 1760. Lambert's ideas were further investigated by August Beer (1853–1932), who published his findings as the Beer–Lambert law in 1851.

Hewlett-Packard ear oximeter

The forerunner of pulse oximetry was the Hewlett-Packard ear oximeter, initially considered to be the "gold standard" against which the first pulse oximeters were compared (Figures 1.1, 1.2).

The Hewlett-Packard ear oximeter uses eight different wavelengths derived from an incandescent source with narrowband interference filters, transmitted to the pinna of the ear by a fibreoptic light guide. Transmitted light leaving the pinna is also led by fibreoptics to the detector. The arterial oxygen saturation is calculated from the absorption over these eight wavelengths. No attempt is made to separate the absorption due to arterial blood from the veins, capillaries, or other tissues. Approximation to arterial saturation is made by heating the ear to cause vasodilation and increase capillary blood flow. The overall absorption then approximates to that of arterial blood. The device has a comparatively large and cumbersome probe-head and needs frequent calibration. It was developed for respiratory physiological study. As it was the only device available for the continuous monitoring of oxygen saturation, the new technique of pulse oximetry was compared with it. As with pulse oximeters, its accuracy was affected by dyshaemoglobins and dyes, despite the use of more than two wavelengths. It was, however, a tremendous advance in oximetry monitoring. Its disadvantages are the very large earpiece, the heavy stiff connection between the earpiece and the main unit, and the necessity for regular calibration.

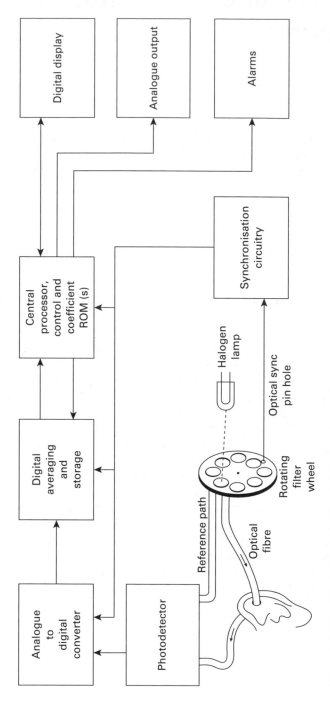

Figure 1.1 Simplified diagram of Hewlett-Packard ear oximeter.

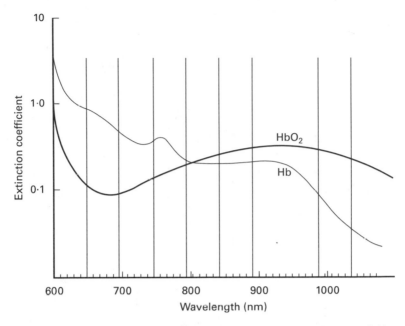

Figure 1.2 Absorption spectra of oxygenated and deoxygenated haemoglobin over wavelengths used in Hewlett-Packard ear oximeter.

Prototype pulse oximeter

The prototype pulse oximeter[1] made use of a halogen incandescent lamp as a light source, and the broad band of energy was passed to a fingertip probe through a glass fibre bundle (Figure 1.3). The transmitted energy was returned to the apparatus by another bundle of fibres. At the apparatus, the returning energy was divided into two paths: one to pass through a narrow bandwidth interference filter centred at 650 nm and the other through a filter centred at 805 nm, an isobestic point for haemoglobin. The energy at the wavelengths selected by each filter was detected by semiconductor sensors, and oxygen saturation was then calculated by analogue computation. There were many disadvantages to this prototype: it had a heavy probe; the fibreoptic cable was unwieldy; unwanted wavelengths passed through the finger, leading to burns; it assumed the Beer–Lambert law but the conditions of the law were not adhered to; it was insensitive with even moderately low pulse pressure; and its analogue electronics were prone to drift.

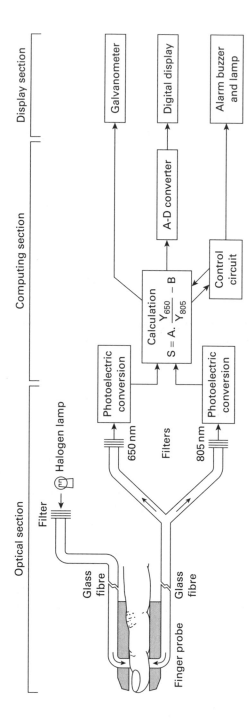

Figure 1.3 Yoshiya's analogue pulse oximeter. Reproduced with permission.[1]

History of pulse oximetry

1851	Beer–Lambert law
1864	Georg Gabriel Stokes discovers a pigment that is the oxygen carrier in blood
1864	Felix Hoppe-Seyler purifies the pigment and calls it haemoglobin
1876	Karl von Veirordt studies the reflection spectra of haemoglobin solutions and the finger
1887–90	Carl Gustav Hufner (1840–84) studies absorption spectra
1919	August Krough (1874–1949) and I Leicht use spectroscopic methods to measure oxygen saturation of blood in fish
1931	Ludwig Nicolai (1904–) investigates the quantitative spectrophotometry of light transmitted through human tissues
1934	Kurt Kramer (1906–85) makes precise measurements of the oxygen saturation of blood flowing through cuvettes
1935	David Drabkin (1899–1980) and James Harold Austin (1883–1952) measure the spectrum of undiluted haemolysed and non-haemolysed blood
1939–45	Second world war: great military interest in oximetry in pilots at high altitude
1940	JR Squires passes red and infrared light through the finger web for the continuous monitoring of oxygenation; it requires compression of tissues to create a bloodless field for calibration
1940–42	Glen Alan Millikan (1906–47) coins the term oximeter and develops the Millikan oximeter
1948–50	Earl Wood (1912–) develops Wood's ear oximeter
1960	Development of the first bench "CO-oximeter" able to distinguish between haemoglobin, carboxyhaemoglobin and methaemoglobin
1964	Robert Shaw develops the eight wavelength ear oximeter
1970	Hewlett-Packard market the eight wavelength ear oximeter
1971	Takuo Aoyagi uses the pulsatility of the absorption signal to separate absorption due to the arteries from the other tissues
1974	Aoyagi develops the prototype pulse oximeter using an incandescent light source, filters, and analogue electronics
1975	First commercially available pulse oximeter

Conventional pulse oximeters

All currently available conventional pulse oximeters use a combination of two wavelengths, normally 660 nm and 940 nm, generated in the probe by combining light-emitting diodes with a miniature semiconductor photodetector, thus providing a compact probe for attachment to the ear or fingertip. A small lightweight cable connects the probe to the main unit. The exception to this arrangement is a pulse oximeter for use in the environment of the magnetic resonance scanner; this oximeter has all of its electronic components in the main unit and the light energy is transmitted to and from the patient by optical fibres.

References

1   Yoshiya I, Shimada Y, Tanaka K. Spectrophotometric monitoring of arterial oxygen saturation at the fingertip. *Med Biol Eng Comput* 1980;**18**: 27–32.

Further reading

Severinghaus JW, Astrup PB. History of blood gas analysis. VI. Oximetry. *J Clin Monit* 1986;**2**:270–88.
Severinghaus JW, Honda Y. History of blood gas analysis. VII. Pulse oximetry. *J Clin Monit* 1987;**3**:135–8.

2: Optical principles

Haemoglobin

Human haemoglobin has a molecular weight of 64 585 daltons and contains two pairs of polypeptide chains: the α-chains have 141 amino acid residues and the β-chains have 146. Each polypeptide chain is combined with one haem group.[1] Each haem group has one atom of iron in the ferrous state and is able to combine reversibly with one molecule of oxygen and yet always be in the ferrous state. To say that haemoglobin consists of four polypeptide chains belies the highly complex three-dimensional shape of the molecule. Figure 2.1 shows the chains in much simplified form.

The amino acid sequence and the positions of the haem groups have been elucidated.[1] The haem groups are attached to the chains through histidine residues by weak bonds and are positioned in crevices in the chains. The quarternary structure of the four chains seems to form a crumpled ball, but the actual shape is of critical importance to pulse oximetry. It not only controls the reaction with oxygen, but the change in the shape of the quarternary structure with level of oxygenation alters the optical absorption spectrum proportionately; this is the basis of optical absorption oximetry.

Spectrophotometry

The concentration of any transparent substance in solution may be measured spectrophotometrically. The components of a simple spectrophotometer are shown in Figure 2.2. Radiant energy is passed through a cuvette of known path length containing the substance under test. The energy source is usually a wide-bandwidth incandescent lamp, and therefore a monochromator is used to produce a single-wavelength monochromatic beam of energy. The monochromator may consist of either a prism, a diffraction grating, or single or multiple narrow-bandwidth interference filter(s). A proportion of the incident energy is absorbed by the solution under test. The Beer–Lambert law relates the fraction of radiant energy absorbed by the substance to the concentration and amount of the substance:

$$A = \log (I_o/I) = \varepsilon l c$$

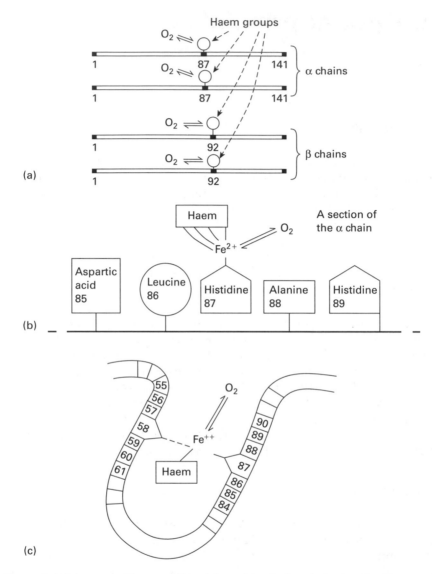

Figure 2.1 Structure of haemoglobin: (a) two identical α chains, each with 141 amino acid residues, and two β chains, each with 146 amino acid residues; (b) attachment of haem group to α chain; (c) crevice containing the haem group. Reproduced with permission of JF Nunn and Butterworth–Heinemann.[2]

A is the absorbence of the sample and is proportional to the concentration (*c*) and the path length (*l*) or depth of the sample. ε is the molar extinction coefficient, which is a wavelength-dependent constant characterising the sample; it is defined as the optical density of an

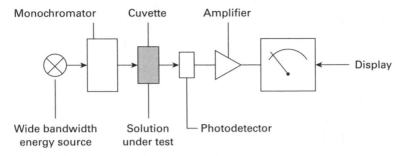

Figure 2.2 Components of a spectrophotometer.

absorbing substance in a concentration of 1 mmol/L measured with a light path length of 1 cm at a specific wavelength. I_o is the intensity of the energy without the sample, and I is the intensity with the sample.

Oximetry by spectrophotometry

Oximetry by any spectrophotometric method relies on the change in colour or, more accurately, in the absorption of electromagnetic energy with change in the percentage of oxygen bound to the haemoglobin molecule. Figure 2.3 shows how the absorption of fully oxygenated and fully deoxygenated adult haemoglobin varies in the wavelength range 400–1000 nm – that is, from the visible light end of the spectrum into the near infrared.

The isobestic points are the wavelengths at which the ε values of two substances, in this case oxygenated and deoxygenated haemoglobin, one of which can be converted into the other, are equal.

It must be remembered, however, that the Beer–Lambert law holds only for monochromatic radiation through a homogeneous and isotropic medium (one in which the refractive index is the same in all directions) with negligible scattering, where there is no association or dissociation of absorbing molecules. There must be a single absorbent, no reaction between the absorbent and the solvent, and no possibility of a photochemical reaction. The only occasion when the conformity of haemoglobin to the Beer–Lambert law may be assumed is for pure aqueous solutions of haemoglobin. Blood is a non-homogeneous liquid which is capable of non-linear absorbance of light, for example as the concentration changes.[3]

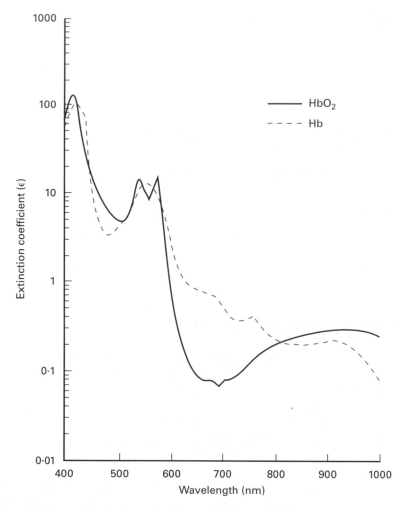

Figure 2.3 Absorption spectra of oxygenated (HbO_2) and deoxygenated (Hb) forms of adult haemoglobin.

Validity of Beer–Lambert Law

Single unknown substance
Clear, non-turbid solution
Constant path length
No photochemical reaction
No reaction between absorbent and solvent

Although the principle of the pulse oximeter relies on the Beer–Lambert law, the above conditions make it clear that, in fact, the

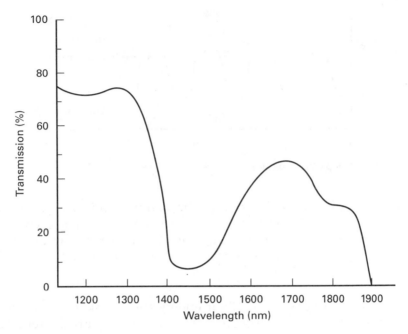

Figure 2.4 Absorption spectrum of distilled water in the near infrared.

calibration of pulse oximetry is empirical, as will be discussed in Chapter 4. This is because of the variable path length, the many different substances in the tissues apart from haemoglobin, and the obvious diffusion, refraction and reflection of the tissues. However, calibration of the pulse oximeter is based on the CO-oximeter, a bench type oximeter in which small samples of heparinised blood are haemolysed and passed into a cuvette of known path length. The CO-oximeter will be described in detail in Chapter 4.

Conventional pulse oximeters function by comparing the absorption of energy at two wavelengths, usually 660 nm and 940 nm, passed through an extremity. A value, SpO_2, which is approximately equal to arterial haemoglobin saturation, SaO_2, is determined from the ratio of the absorption of the energy at the two wavelengths. The range of wavelengths over which spectrophotometric techniques can be used *in vivo* is limited to a "window" of between 600 and 1300 nm. At wavelengths shorter than 600 nm red skin pigment (melanin) causes a high level of absorption, whereas at wavelengths longer than 1300 nm there is strong absorption owing to the water in the tissues (Figure 2.4).

The light sources – light-emitting diodes – are placed in close contact with one skin surface. The light energy is detected with a

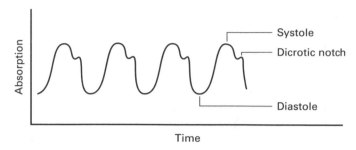

Figure 2.5 Photoplethysmogram.

semiconductor detector, placed on the skin perpendicularly opposite the diodes in the case of the transmittance pulse oximeter. A few pulse oximeters, including those used in fetal pulse oximetry, rely on a reflected signal and therefore have the detector mounted adjacent to the light-emitting diodes.

The interaction between the light energy and the skin, other tissues and blood is complex. The incident energy is partially reflected, remitted (diffuse reflectance), refracted, absorbed and scattered. Without this complex interaction between the light energy and the tissues neither transmission nor reflectance pulse oximetry could work, except through the earlobe. This is because remittance (diffuse reflectance) is obviously required for reflectance pulse oximetry, and diffraction is required to bypass the bone in transmission pulse oximetry.

There are many structures, entities or chemical compounds in the tissues of the extremity on which the pulse oximeter is applied that absorb at the same wavelengths as the haemoglobin of arterial blood. However, owing to the cardiac rhythm, the absorption of light due to the haemoglobin in the arteries and arterioles increases during systole and decreases during diastole (Figure 2.5).

In practice, the light absorption through the finger varies by about 1–2% of the total absorption. This is not entirely due to the increase in diameter of the arteries and arterioles during systole: if it were, then the variation in absorption during the cardiac cycle would be very much less. A pulse oximeter will operate satisfactorily when the probe is placed on a rigid, transparent tube through which blood is passing in a pulsatile flow. A photoplethysmogram of such a system will show the pulsatility.

Examination of the fluid mechanics of blood shows that the axis of the erythrocytes changes during the cardiac cycle (Figure 2.6). During

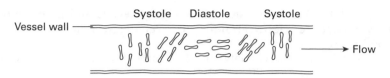

Figure 2.6 Changes in axis of erythrocytes during cardiac cycle.

diastole they tend to align their major diameter parallel to the direction of flow, whereas during systole their major diameter aligns perpendicular to the flow, thereby presenting a greater absorption path length.[4] The change in erythrocyte axis also contributes to the change in reflectance during the cardiac cycle, which is important in the reflection mode of pulse oximetry. This theory is also supported by the electrical conductance of blood in motion, which changes (as does the optical reflectance and transmittance) with any change in the velocity of blood flow.[5]

In attempts to increase the accuracy of pulse oximetry and to reduce the delays between changes in actual SaO_2 and the indicated SpO_2 value, experimental reflection-type pulse oximeter probes have been applied more centrally. Probes were applied to the left tracheal mucosa with variation of SpO_2 value, depending upon the pressure of application.[6] The accuracy was greater with a cuff pressure of 10–60 cmH_2O than when it was around zero, suggesting that the readings may not be primarily derived from the mucosa but from deeper tissues.

Another site where the application of the probe may prove easier is the pharynx. This has been shown to produce accurate results in low perfusion states. The probe was attached to a laryngeal mask airway.[7,8]

Agro et al.[9] also found that the application pressure using a laryngeal mask airway did not affect the accuracy.

References

1 Perutz MF. The haemoglobin molecule. *Proc Roy Soc* 1969;**B173**:113–40.
2 Nunn JF. *Applied respiratory physiology, 3rd edn.* London: Butterworths, 1987.
3 Wukitsch MW, Petterson MT, Tobler DR, Pologe JA. Pulse oximetry: analysis of theory, technology, and practice. *J Clin Monit* 1988;**4**:290–301.
4 Nijboer JA, Dorlas JC, Mahieu HF. Photoelectric plethysmography – some fundamental aspects of the reflection and transmission method. *Clin Phys Physiol Meas* 1981;**7**:205–15.

5 Visser KR, Lamberts R, Korsten HHM, Zijlstra WG. Observations on blood flow related to electrical impedance changes. *Pflugers Arch* 1976; **366**:289–91.
6 Brimacombe J, Keller C, Margreiter J. A pilot study of left tracheal pulse oximetry. *Anesth Analg* 2000;**91**:1003–6.
7 Brimacombe J, Keller C. Successful pharyngeal pulse oximetry in low perfusion states. *Can J Anaesth* 2000;**47**:907.
8 Keller C, Brimacombe J, Agro F, Margreiter J. A pilot study of pharyngeal pulse oximetry with the laryngeal mask airway: a comparison with finger oximetry and arterial saturation measurements in healthy anaesthetised patients. *Anesth Analg* 2000;**90**:440–4.
9 Agro F, Carassiti M, Cataldo R, Ghherardi S, Barzoi G. Pulse oximetry with the laryngeal mask airway. *Resuscitation* 1999;**43**:65–7.

3: How pulse oximetry works

Chapter 1 described how the absorption of light energy by haemoglobin varies with the level of oxygenation. The pulse oximeter has to separate this change in absorbance due to varying oxygenation from all the other absorbents when the device is used on the human extremity. The pulse oximeter performs spectrophotometry either by reflection from the skin and subcutaneous tissues or, more commonly, by transmission through an extremity. Most pulse oximeters currently in use are of the transmission type, although for special purposes, for example intrapartum monitoring, the reflection technique is used. As transmission pulse oximetry is the most common method in use, this will be discussed first.

The extremity chosen – usually the finger (or occasionally a toe, the earlobe or the bridge of the nose) – needs to have a reasonably short optical path length to be sufficiently translucent at the wavelengths used. The wavelengths used must be chosen to be within the "window" between 600 nm and 1300 nm. They must also be at wavelengths on the absorption spectrum where the two species of haemoglobin have widely different absorptions (Figure 3.1). Knowledge of simultaneous equations dictates that the minimum number of wavelengths used must be equal to or greater than the number of unknowns; therefore, conventional pulse oximetry makes use of two wavelengths, as there are two unknowns – namely, oxygenated haemoglobin and deoxygenated haemoglobin.

For the design of suitable equipment, wavelengths must be chosen which are easy to generate, ideally monochromatic, and low in cost. A sufficiently sensitive detector is also required so that high energy levels, which may cause tissue damage, are not needed. Finally, pulse oximetry requires some computing power to extract a saturation value for arterial haemoglobin from all the other absorbents in the optical path.

Spectrophotometry requires monochromatic energy sources, that is, energy of a single "colour" or single wavelength. The only device that comes anywhere near this specification is the laser. If lasers were used for pulse oximetry, it would be necessary to use two lasers of different wavelengths and to guide the energy to the patient's extremity via optical fibres. This would make pulse oximeters very expensive and fragile, and have safety implications.

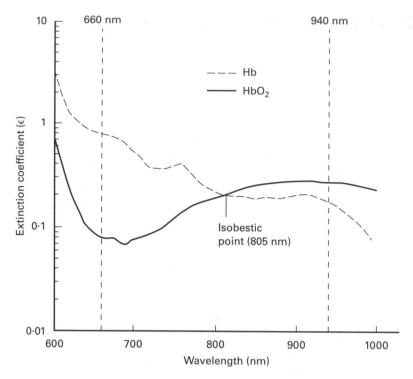

Figure 3.1 Absorption spectra of oxygenated and deoxygenated haemoglobin, showing the two most commonly used wavelengths.

Mass production of pulse oximeters became possible when it was realised that light-emitting diodes (LED), although not strictly monochromatic, could be used as a suitable energy source. This makes the fibreoptic light cable unnecessary and also reduces the risk of overheating the tissues. With a separate energy source (LED) for each wavelength, it also becomes unnecessary to use narrow-bandwidth interference filters, which are delicate and expensive. LEDs can also be switched on and off very rapidly, as they do not have the thermal inertia of incandescent (heated filament) energy sources. Thus it is possible to use a single photodetector if the LEDs are rapidly switched alternately on and off.

Probe

Light-emitting diodes

A semiconductor junction diode is a device that allows an electric current to pass in one direction only.[1] The junction in the minute piece of silicon from which the diode is manufactured is produced by "doping" the silicon with minuscule amounts of impurities such as aluminium, gallium or indium. Ordinary silicon semiconductor diodes emit energy when current is passed in the forward direction; this energy is at about 1100 nm and the device is designed to minimise this wasted energy. However, by "doping" the semiconductor with carefully chosen mixtures of impurities, it is possible to produce diodes that emit energy at other wavelengths. Further, the design of the diode is optimised for energy emission.

Ideally the energy sources used in pulse oximetry should be monochromatic, that is, of only one wavelength or of an infinitely narrow bandwidth. It is possible to produce energy sources of exceedingly narrow bandwidth in the form of semiconductor lasers, but these are also very expensive by comparison.

The early generations of pulse oximeters all used similar wavelengths, namely 660 nm (red) and 940 nm (near infrared). However, modern devices, including transmission, reflection and intrauterine pulse oximeters, often make use of other wavelengths. LEDs of 660 nm and 940 nm were originally chosen, as they were wavelengths that were easy to manufacture, but a much greater range of wavelengths is now available (see Box).

Gallium arsenide doping of the semiconductor material of light-emitting diodes to produce specific wavelengths

Ultraviolet	455–350 nm	GaN GaS2
Violet	455–390 nm	GaN
Blue	492–455 nm	GaAs-phosphor (ZnS, SiC)
Green	577–492 nm	GaP:N
Yellow	597–577 nm	GaAs.14P.86
Orange	622–597 nm	GaAs.35P.65
Red	780–622 nm	GaP:ZnO GaAs.6P.4
Near infrared	810 nm	GaAlAs
	880 nm	GaAlAs
	900 nm	GaAs
	940 nm	GaAsSi
	1100 nm	Ga.17In.83As.34P.66
Infrared	1250 nm	Ga.28In.72As.6P.4

Conventional pulse oximetry requires the use of one wavelength each side of the 805 nm isobestic point on the absorption spectra of adult haemoglobin (Figure 3.1). The choice of the near infrared LED at 940 nm was easy, as the absorption spectra are reasonably flat at this wavelength so that slight variations in the peak wavelength will make

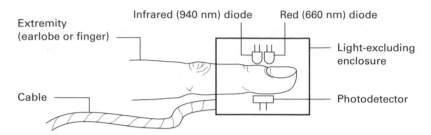

Figure 3.2 Components of transmission pulse oximeter probe.

very little difference to calibration. The advantage of 660 nm as the red wavelength chosen is that there is a comparatively large difference in the absorption between reduced and oxygenated haemoglobin at this point on the spectrum, yielding detectable changes in absorption with small changes in oxygen saturation. Although the curves are not horizontal at 660 nm, they are considerably flatter than at shorter wavelengths.

Advantages of light-emitting diodes over other energy sources:

- Narrow bandwidth (almost monochromatic)
- High efficiency
- Low temperature
- High switching speed (>1 MHz)
- Stable peak wavelength
- Intensity varies linearly with drive current
- Inexpensive compared with alternatives (semiconductor lasers)
- Safer than semiconductor lasers.

The probe of a conventional pulse oximeter consists of the energy sources in the form of light-emitting diodes, mounted in such a way that their output is directed perpendicularly through the extremity to a semiconductor photodetector. This is shown diagrammatically in Figure 3.2, but it is important that it is a snug fit, with a constant but light pressure on the tissues, and that the energy cannot bypass the tissues. The whole assembly must be protected from extraneous light over the range of wavelengths to which the detector is sensitive.

The mechanical design of the probe must also ensure that the position of the probe is correct and remains so, as malpositioning may upset its calibration, especially with small children.[2]

Manufacturers are now paying more attention to electrical screening of the probe assembly and using differential amplifier techniques in the

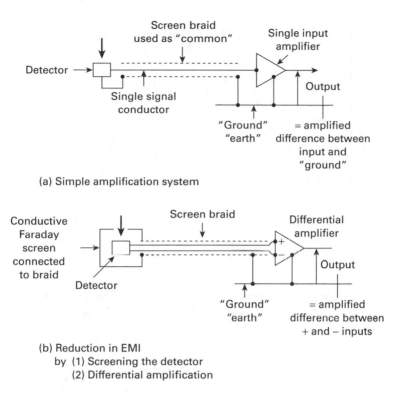

(a) Simple amplification system

(b) Reduction in EMI
by (1) Screening the detector
(2) Differential amplification

Figure 3.3 Electronic reduction in interference at the probe.

amplification of the plethysmograph signal to reduce the common-mode electrical and magnetic noise. The simplest way of amplifying a small signal is shown in Figure 3.3a, where there is one signal conductor and the other current pathway is the "common", which is often the screening braid of the flexible cable from the probe to the unit. If electromagnetic interference (EMI) affects the probe or the lead it will affect the signal conductor slightly differently from the "common". With the very small signal voltages involved, the voltage generated by the EMI may even be greater than the signal itself. Using a differential amplifier (Figure 3.3b), there are two identical conductors from the detector to an amplifier whose output is a function of the difference between these two conductors. Any EMI affecting these two signal leads will induce identical voltages, which therefore cancel each other out. This is an important technique used in any small-signal medical application (e.g. ECG, EEG, EMG, direct BP etc.).

As there are great variations in the thickness and pigmentation of the finger, the energy output of the LEDs must be variable to achieve an output from the photodetector that does not vary greatly with the

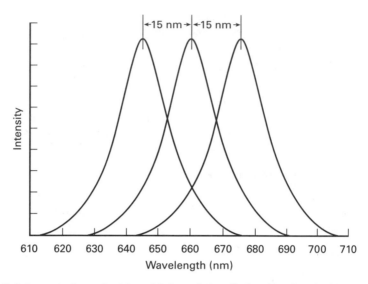

Figure 3.4 Spread of wavelengths of light-emitting diodes. Reprinted with permission from *International Anesthesiology Clinics*, vol. 25, pp. 137–153, 1987.

overall density or thickness of the finger. This is so that the energy levels reaching the semiconductor detector are always detectable and yet never overload or saturate it. It is also important that unnecessarily high levels of energy are not inflicted on the tissues, which would otherwise suffer heat damage. The intensity of the output of the LED may be varied over several orders of magnitude by varying the current passing through it while it is switched on.

Light-emitting diodes do have some disadvantages as the energy source for pulse oximetry. They have a bandwidth of between 10 and 50 nm, depending upon their centre or peak wavelength. Owing to production spreads, there is a variation in the centre wavelength of different diodes of the same type. In fact, no two samples are exactly the same,[3] and there may be a variation of up to 15 nm either side of the centre wavelength (Figure 3.4).

A similar variation may occur with variation of the driving current.[4] This is of little consequence with the near infrared LED, as the absorption spectra in this region are flat, whereas small variations in the centre wavelength of the red LED will cause comparatively large errors as the curves are steeper in this region (Figure 3.1). The designer may cope with this problem in one of three ways: by carefully selecting from each batch of LEDs only those that are within an acceptable range of error from the chosen centre wavelength; or by measuring the centre wavelength of each LED used and adjusting the calibration of the pulse oximeter to take account of the actual wavelength; or the problem may be ignored. If the range of error is ignored, the pulse oximeter may be inaccurate if its probe has a red LED at the extreme of the tolerance set by the manufacturer. This inaccuracy will increase as the oxygen saturation decreases. So that probes of the same type are interchangeable between different examples of the same pulse oximeter, some manufacurers have a preset calibration component, usually in the form of a fixed resistor mounted in the connector of the probe lead. This calibration resistor is set by the manufacturer when the probe is made, to correspond to the red LED wavelength. When the probe is connected to the oximeter, the calibration of the device is automatically corrected for the wavelength of that particular probe.

Photodetector

A single photodetector is used to detect the energy alternately from both LEDs. In conventional transmission pulse oximetry, it is positioned perpendicular opposite the LEDs with the extremity snugly held between them (Figure 3.2). This assembly must be protected from extraneous light over the range of wavelengths to which the detector is sensitive.

In the case of transmission pulse oximetry, the photodetector is mounted a small but discrete distance away from and in the same plane as the LEDs. The photodetector is usually a silicon photodiode. Most semiconductors alter their electrical properties when exposed to outside energy; this is considered to be a disadvantage, and semiconductor manufacturers go to enormous lengths to avoid this problem. Semiconductor photodetectors, however, take advantage of this property. Photosensitivity is usually over a limited bandwidth, and this limits the selection of device and the range of wavelengths of LEDs in a particular case. The silicon photodiode has a large dynamic range, with a linear change in its output proportional to incident light level over a range of 10 decades of light energy. Phototransistors are more sensitive than photodiodes but have the disadvantage of being electrically more "noisy".[5] Furthermore, the sensitivity of all photodetectors varies with wavelength, and it is necessary to take this into account in the design of the electronics and in calibration.

The flexible cable from the probe to the pulse oximeter unit carries the power to the LEDs and the signal from the photodetector. This signal may be extremely small, so the cable needs to be electrically screened; the conductors of the power and the signal are therefore surrounded by a flexible conductive braid "screening" to protect them from electromagnetic interference. The cable may also contain conductors for a temperature sensor, which detects the temperature of the probe and the underlying skin. The cable needs to be flexible and light, so that reasonable movement will not cause mechanically induced artefacts of the probe.

Electronics

The main unit of the pulse oximeter contains electronic circuitry with functions listed in the Box.

Electronic functions in the pulse oximeter

- Amplification of the photodetector signal
- Separation of the red and infrared plethysmograph signals
- Switching and control of current through light-emitting diodes
- Adjustment of the gain of one of the two signals to make them equivalent
- Separation of the "arterial" component of the signal
- Analogue-to-digital conversion of the red and infrared signals
- Calculation of the red:infrared ratio
- Reduction or elimination of artefacts
- "Calculation" of the oxygen saturation (SpO_2)
- Display:

    SpO_2
    plethysmogram
    heart rate

- Control of alarms
- Storage of trend of SpO_2

The signal in either the red or the infrared channels is due to the absorption of some of the energy during its transit from LED to photodetector. This absorption is made up of a number of components, as shown in Figure 3.5.

Figure 3.6 shows the electronics. Although the initial stage of amplification is by conventional analogue electronics and the "calculation" of the oxygen saturation (SpO_2) is always carried out digitally with a microprocessor, the photodetector signal may be processed in between by either analogue or digital techniques. At the point in the system where digital electronics takes over, the signal or signals are converted by an analogue-to-digital converter (ADC) to a form suitable for manipulation by the microprocessor.

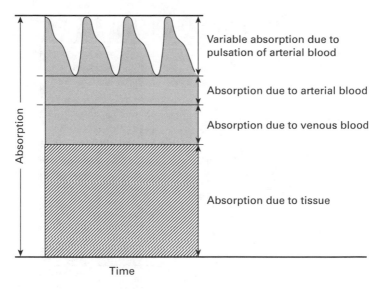

Figure 3.5 Components of absorption signal.

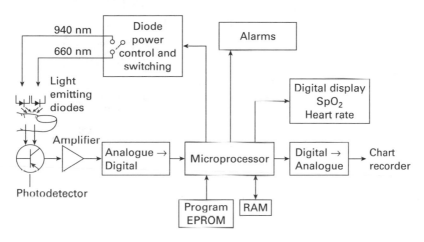

Figure 3.6 Electronic components of pulse oximeter.

The incoming signal from the photodetector is of very low amplitude and is first amplified. The light-emitting diodes are energised alternately, but it is usual to introduce a short period when neither is energised, so that any extraneous ambient light may be measured. The amplified signal is then split into three components – red, infrared, and a signal equivalent to the "dark" or ambient light period. When these signals are passed through electronic filters, the

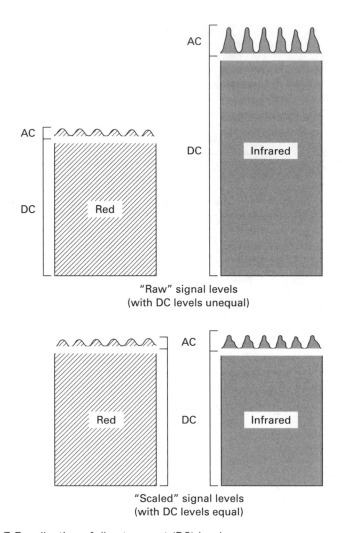

"Raw" signal levels
(with DC levels unequal)

"Scaled" signal levels
(with DC levels equal)

Figure 3.7 Equalisation of direct current (DC) levels.

high-frequency (1 kHz) switching is removed so that the signals appear as though they each come from a continuous source of each wavelength. The level of ambient light detected during the dark period is subtracted from the levels of direct current (DC) to avoid any error caused by this source of energy. One of the two photoplethysmograph signals is next altered in amplitude until the DC components of the red and infrared signals are equal (Figure 3.7). It is then possible to calculate the ratio of red to infrared of the amplitudes of the alternating current (AC) components.

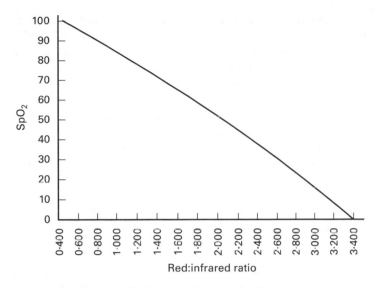

Figure 3.8 Relation between SpO$_2$ and red:infrared ratio.

Early pulse oximeters compared the amplitude ratio between the components of the red and infrared signals once each cardiac cycle. In later-generation pulse oximeters, improved accuracy is obtained by calculating the ratio many times each cardiac cycle.

It may be considered that accurate values of SpO$_2$ can be obtained by the simple application of simultaneous equations describing the Beer–Lambert law, but this is not the case. As mentioned in Chapter 2, the Beer–Lambert law only applies under certain conditions, namely a single unknown, no scattering or turbidity, and a constant path length. Many pulse oximeters apply the "red:infrared ratio" to a "look-up table". The relations between oxygen saturation and the red:infrared ratio is shown in Figure 3.8.

Algorithms are also employed to input light intensity as a variable, and also continuous small variations in the thickness of path length.

The reader is referred to a complementary text written for engineers and physicists for further in-depth discussion of the technicalities of the algorithms used (see Further reading).

There is a large variation in optical density from patient to patient, owing to the size and thickness of the finger (or earlobe) and to skin pigmentation. Although the dynamic range of the silicon photodiode is large, saturation of this semiconductor device would occur if the same intensity of light were applied to a small child as to a large, heavily pigmented man. There would also be a risk of causing heat damage to the child's tissues. For these reasons, the LED current is adjusted by controlled steps until the minimum light energy is received by the photodetector for accurate calculation of SpO_2. The intensities of the two light-emitting diodes must be adjusted in synchronism. This control of the current through the diode is another function of the microprocessor. The microprocessor must introduce a correction factor to the calibration with changes in diode current because of the small variations in peak wavelength mentioned previously.

Elimination of artefacts

If the user were presented with saturation values exactly as they were calculated, the displayed value could be continuously changing at the rate at which the values were being calculated. These values would also include some that were invalid, as they were generated by artefacts. For this reason, statistical averaging techniques are included in the software.

The first requirement is to try to eliminate artefacts caused by mechanical movement. The algorithm used by Nellcor in their most modern range of pulse oximeters is shown in Figure 3.9.

Different manufacturers use different averaging methods. Ohmeda use a weighted averaging scheme, which takes into account the magnitude of the instantaneous signal, the point in the cardiac cycle at which the relevant data were taken, and the correlation of the instantaneous value of saturation with the current displayed average value. If the new instantaneous value of saturation is very different from the displayed value it is assigned a low weighting. A running average of those weighted values is maintained for a period of the previous 3 seconds. Thus short sharp aberrations in measured saturation are "ironed out", but during periods of actual rapidly changing saturation all the weights will tend to be reduced, thereby facilitating rapid response and close tracking of the arterial oxygen saturation.[6]

The Masimo Corporation have developed and patented the Masimo-SET® or Signal Extraction Technology. Here the software maps a time series of detected plethysmographic information into a plot of possible saturation values (x axis) versus the probability that such values exist in the time series (y axis). During periods without

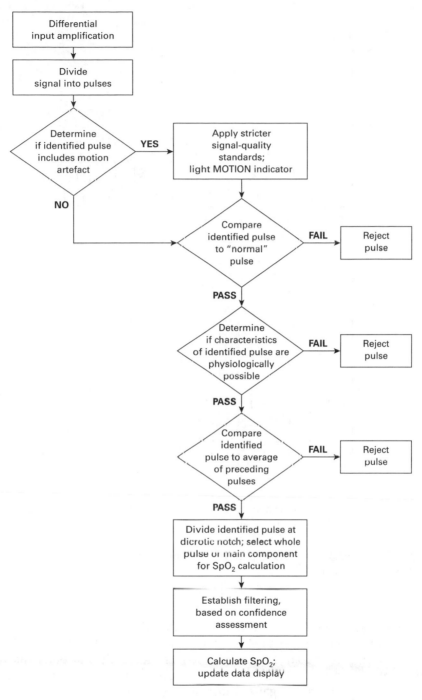

Figure 3.9 Overview of Nellcor OXISMART advanced signal-processing technology. Reproduced with permission of Nellcor Corporation, USA.

(a)

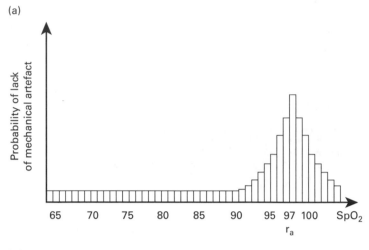

(b)

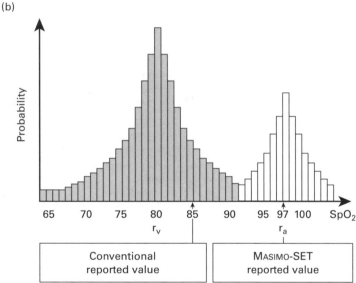

Figure 3.10 Principle of Masimo-SET artefact elimination. (By kind permission of Masimo Corporation.)

mechanical artefacts being generated, when the "noise" contribution is therefore small, the saturation value has a high probability of being accurate (Figure 3.10a). During periods of mechanical artefact many different saturation values may be calculated, but the software is able to use the information gained during the period of no mechanical artefact to select the SpO_2 value with the highest probability of being correct (Figure 3.10b).

Improved design of the sensor technology has also contributed to reductions in mechanical and EMI artefacts.

Status messages

Apart from displays of saturation, heart rate and plethysmograph, most pulse oximeters also display messages:

"no probe connected" "probe off patient"
"noise signal" "searching for pulse"
"battery low" "insufficient signal".

Alarms

All pulse oximeters must have alarms for low saturation and for low and high heart rate. Many also have an alarm for high oxygen saturation, but this should be deprecated: this high saturation alarm is provided for use in neonatal medicine, when the pulse oximeter is used instead of transcutaneous oxygen partial pressure monitoring (discussed in Chapter 12).

The alarms on pulse oximeters should automatically be set to default values when the device is switched on. Common default values are $SpO_2 < 95\%$ and heart rate 60–100 beats/min. These levels can be adjusted by the user but must reset to the default values when the pulse oximeter is switched off.

Another useful warning provided by some manufacturers, although under the patent control of one manufacturer, is a change in the audible frequency of the pulse beep. A decrease in the frequency of the beep very quickly alerts the user to a fall in oxygen saturation.

Trending

Many pulse oximeters provide a software recording facility, automatically plotting the saturation over periods of one, two, six or 12 hours displayed as a graph on the display normally used for the plethysmogram. Some pulse oximeters also have a facility for direct recording of the saturation and heart rate on a chart recorder or with a computer. These facilities are especially useful in sleep studies for obstructive sleep apnoea.

Power supply

The pulse oximeter obviously needs a power supply. Any consideration of the source of power must include whether or not it will be necessary to use the device away from mains electricity, and if so, for how long. The internal power requirements of the pulse oximeter may be considered in three sections: the light-emitting diodes; the "electronics"; and the displays.

The diodes require between 10 mA and 200 mA, depending on the overall density of the tissues through which they are having to transmit the energy. However, they usually have a duty ratio (ratio of time-on to time-off) of 1:3 for each diode, so that each is on for one-third of the time.

The "electronics", which includes the preamplifiers, the analogue-to-digital converter and the microprocessor, may be designed to use conventional integrated circuits or with very low-current components. Not all pulse oximeters are designed with very low-current devices. This is because the very low-current integrated circuits are generally more delicate to work with, are more susceptible to static electricity, and are more expensive. It is also easier to achieve very high-speed calculations with the higher-current integrated circuits.

A wide variety of display methods is available to the pulse oximeter designer, each with its own advantages and disadvantages. The cathode ray tube display is the most versatile but has the highest current requirements. A low voltage of around 6 V at approximately 100 mA is needed to energise the filament that is the source of free electrons in the cathode ray tube, but the greatest amount of power is required to generate the extra high tension of between 5 kV and 10 kV to accelerate the electrons from the filament to the phosphor screen. Although only a few milliamperes are required at this extra high tension, its generation is inefficient.

Seven-segment LED displays are the most visible at a distance and from wide angles. These displays require only a few volts, but at a comparatively high current; the higher the current, the greater the intensity. Liquid crystal displays require very low current to control them, but they are less legible than light-emitting diode displays. Legibility is greatly improved by lighting from behind, but this back-lighting has a comparatively high current consumption. Display technology is still in its infancy, and developments are rapidly being made.

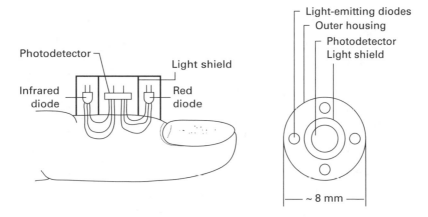

Figure 3.11 Section (left) and plan (right) of reflection oximeter probe.

In summary, it would be difficult to reduce the power requirements of the light-emitting diodes in the probe, but the requirements of the electrons and the display are a compromise between legibility and portability. The more portable pulse oximeters contain either sealed lead acid secondary cell batteries, nickel–cadmium, or nickel–metal hydride batteries. Battery chargers are provided and should be internal rather than a separate item. (Battery chargers for lead acid and nickel–cadmium batteries are not interchangeable.)

Reflection pulse oximetry

There are certain advantages in using reflected rather than trans-mitted light. The design of the probe is simpler, with greater mechanical strength (Figure 3.11).

From a clinical point of view a reflection pulse oximeter has the advantage that it can be used at more sites than the transmission type, for example the forearm, thigh, chest, forehead and cheeks. This means that its saturation readings can be made in patients with poorer perfusion and in those who are hypothermic. The reflection pulse oximeter may prove useful after cardiac bypass surgery, where initially the periphery is very shut down and much cooler than normal. Palve[7] showed that saturation could be measured with a reflection-type probe from a patient's forehead when the fingertip temperature was only 28·8°C. Reflection pulse oximetry works well on ventilated patients who are unconscious, but difficulty with probe

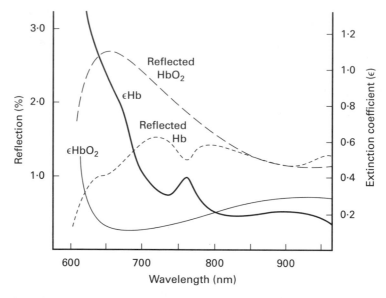

Figure 3.12 Comparison of absorption and reflection spectra of oxygenated (HbO$_2$) and deoxygenated (Hb) haemoglobin (from data of Zijlstra and Mook[10]).

fixation may lead to more mechanical artefact problems with conscious or restless patients.[8]

The accuracy of reflection pulse oximetry may sometimes be poorer than by transmission; this may be due to lower signal-to-noise ratio, smaller heart-related pulsations, and less reliable electronic signal analysis.[9] Compared to transmission pulse oximetry a smaller fraction of the illuminated light reaches the photodetector. Wavelengths are similar to the transmission mode, although one manufacturer has used the isobestic wavelength 805 nm.

Tissue oedema also reduces the sensitivity of reflection pulse oximetry. Other uses include the assessment of the blood supply of skin flaps and other transplanted organs, and of the viability of injured extremities and organs. In these applications the reflection probe must be placed in a sterile plastic sleeve.

The reflection spectra of oxygenated and deoxygenated blood are shown in Figure 3.12. There is a resemblance to the absorption spectra shown in Figure 3.1. The electronics and display of the reflection pulse oximeter are identical to those of the transmission pulse oximeter.

The pulse oximeter and magnetic resonance imaging

The very high magnetic field strengths involved in magnetic resonance imaging (MRI) make the use of conventional electronic monitoring equipment impossible. The problem is due to voltages being induced in any conductor being moved in a "permanent" magnetic field, and to the radiofrequency magnetic pulses generated in that magnetic field. These voltages not only upset the monitoring equipment but may permanently damage it. Any metal connection to the skin of the patient also lead to burns. Metal conductors in the MRI scanner also cause distortion of the images.

To overcome this problem some manufacturers have produced pulse oximeters especially for use with the MRI scanner. All of the electronic components, including the light-emitting diodes and the photodetector, are in the housing of the main unit. The light energy is then directed to and from the patient by optical fibres. The magnetic field affects the passage of light along the optical fibre, but only by an infinitesimal amount compared to the amplitude of the plethysmograph and oximetry signals. Such pulse oximeters have been assessed and found to operate successfully and safely,[11] but as the main unit of the pulse oximeter contains ferromagnetic components the pulse oximeter must be kept at least 3 m away from the bore of the MRI magnet.

References

1 Sze SM. *The physics of semiconductor devices*. Chichester: John Wiley & Sons, 1981.
2 Barker SJ, Hyatt J, Shah NK, Kao YJ. The effect of sensor malpositioning on pulse oximeter accuracy during hypoxia. *Anesthesiology* 1993;**79**:248-54.
3 Pologe JA. Pulse oximetry: technical aspects. *Int Anesthesiol Clin* 1987;**25**:137-53.
4 de Kock JP, Reynolds KJ, Tarassenko L, Moyle JTB. The effect of varying LED intensity on pulse oximeter accuracy. *J Med Eng Technol* 1991;**15**: 111-15.
5 Burke MJ, Whelan MV. Photoplethysmography: selecting optoelectronic components. *Med Biol Eng Comput* 1986;**24**:647-50.
6 Wukitsch MW, Petterson MT, Tobler DR, Pologe JA. Pulse oximetry: analysis of theory, technology, and practice. *J Clin Monit* 1988;**4**:290-301.
7 Palve H. Comparison of reflection and transmission pulse oximetry after open heart surgery. *Crit Care Med* 1992;**20**:48-51.
8 Cheng EY, Hopwood MB, Kay J. Forehead pulse oximetry compared with finger pulse oximetry and arterial blood gas measurement. *J Clin Monit* 1987;**4**:223-6.

9   Takatani S, Davies C, Sakakibara N. Experimental and clinical evaluation of a non-invasive reflectance pulse oximeter sensor. *J Clin Monit* 1992;**8**: 257–66.

10 Zijlstra WG, Mook GA. *Medical reflection photometry*. Assen, The Netherlands: Van Gorcum, 1962.

11 Shellock FG, Myers SM, Kimble KJ. Monitoring heart rate and oxygen saturation with a fibreoptic pulse oximeter during MR imaging. *Am J Roentgenol* 1991;**158**:663–4.

Further reading

Webster JG (ed). *Design of pulse oximeters*, Medical Science Series. Institute of Physics Publishing, 1997.

4: Calibration

The first pulse oximeters were calibrated by using a theoretical approach based on the Beer–Lambert law:

$$OD = \log (I_o/I) = \varepsilon c d$$

where OD is the optical density, I_o is incident light, I is transmitted light, ε is the extinction coefficient, c is the concentration of the sample and d is the optical path length.

As stated in Chapter 2, the Beer–Lambert law applies only under conditions of non-turbidity, a single unknown solute and a fixed optical path length. None of these conditions pertains in clinical pulse oximetry.[1] All manufacturers have abandoned the calculation of saturation by the Beer–Lambert law and use empirical data for calibration.

Until recently, calibration of pulse oximeters was by *in vivo* comparison with discrete samples of arterial blood analysed with a CO-oximeter. Currently, several groups are working on *in vitro* calibration by using human blood in an artificial circulation.[2] Others have developed methods of checking the calibration of pulse oximeters using non-haem methods.

It is, firstly, most important to define what the pulse oximeter actually measures and indicates. There is much argument as to whether pulse oximeters are calibrated to measure functional or fractional oxygen saturation. These two definitions are derived from the historical methods of measurement of oxygen carried by blood. The van Slyke method measured the actual volume of oxygen per unit volume of blood.[3] This was compared with the oxygen capacity, which was the volume of oxygen carried by an identical sample of blood after it had been equilibrated with room air. Historically, oxygen saturation was defined as the content as a percentage of the capacity. By this definition of oxygen saturation, any forms of haemoglobin in the sample that do not bind oxygen in a reversible way are not included. Thus any carboxyhaemoglobin or methaemoglobin in the sample was excluded. This is now referred to as functional haemoglobin saturation:

$$\text{Functional SaO}_2 = \frac{\text{HbO}_2}{\text{HbO}_2 + \text{Hb}} \times 100\%$$

Modern multiwavelength spectrophotometers can measure all four common species of haemoglobin (haemoglobin A, oxygenated haemoglobin, carboxyhaemoglobin, and methaemoglobin). The percentage oxygen saturation of the haemoglobin is now defined as a ratio of the amount of haemoglobin saturated with oxygen to all the four species. This is termed the fractional saturation:

$$\text{Fractional SaO}_2 = \frac{\text{HbO}_2}{\text{HbO}_2 + \text{Hb} + \text{HbCO} + \text{MetHb}} \times 100\%$$

Ideally, the pulse oximeter should measure either fractional or functional saturation, and the manufacturer should state whether a particular unit has been calibrated as fractional or functional. However, with current pulse oximeters using only two wavelengths, it must be said that pulse oximeters indicate neither functional nor fractional saturation.[4] The conventional two-wavelength pulse oximeter measures the absorption at two wavelengths and applies their ratio to look-up tables, which then indicate a value, SpO_2, which is best defined as *oxygen saturation as measured by a pulse oximeter.*

The blood gas analyser has electrodes that measure the partial pressures of oxygen and carbon dioxide, and also the concentration of hydrogen ions in the plasma. The oxygen is usually measured with a Clark polarographic electrode, and the carbon dioxide by a Severinghaus electrode. These measurements are displayed as such, but most blood gas analysers also display oxygen saturation (SO_2). This value of saturation is derived from the measured oxygen pressure (PO_2), taking into account the effects of carbon dioxide pressure (PCO_2), pH and temperature, and also assuming healthy adult human haemoglobin. Even when all the factors have been taken into account, it is still not possible to calculate accurately the percentage oxygen saturation, as witnessed by the different algorithms currently in use,[5] some of which are shown in the Box on p. 37. The reason for this inaccuracy is the necessity of predicting the exact shape and any shift of the oxyhaemoglobin dissociation curve for a particular blood sample. The effects of changes in pH, temperature, and the partial pressure of carbon dioxide on the oxyhaemoglobin dissociation curve are discussed in Chapter 6.

Equations for determining oxygen saturation

Heck[6]

$$SO_2 = 100/(1 + 10^{-(\log PO_2 - 0.48\,PH - 0.0013\,BE - 4.962)/0.369})\%$$

Kelman[7]

$$SO_2 = 100 \cdot (a_1x + a_2x^2 + a_3x^3 + x^4)/(a_4 + a_5x + a_6x^2 + a_7x^2 + x^4)\%$$
$$x = pO_2 \cdot 10^{(0.0024(37-TEMP) - 0.40\,(PH - 7.40) + 0.06\,(\log 40 - \log PCO_2))}$$

$a_1 = -8.5322289 \cdot 10^5$
$a_2 = 2.1214010 \cdot 10^3$
$a_3 = -6 \times 7073989 \cdot 10$
$a_4 = 9.3596087 \cdot 10^5$
$a_5 = -3.1346258 \cdot 10^4$
$a_6 = 2.3961674 \cdot 10^3$
$a_7 = -6.7104406 \cdot 10$

Lutz[8,9]

$$SO_2 = 100/((26.7/pO_{2ST})^{2.7} + 1)\%$$
$$pO_{2ST} = pO_{2AC} \cdot 10^{0.48\,(PHAC - 7.4) + 0.0013\,BE}$$
pO_{2ST} = standard pO_2
pO_{2AC} = actual pO_2

Marsoner[10]

$$SO_2 = Q/(Q + 1)\%$$
$$\log Q = -4.14 + 1.661 \cdot exp_{10}(-0.074 \cdot pO_2) + 2.9 \cdot \log pO_2$$
$$+ \log (1 + 10^{PH - 6.81}) - \log (1 + 10^{8.03 - PH})$$

Severinghaus[11]

$$SO_2 = (((pO_2 \cdot e^{1.1(PH - 7.4)})^3 + 150 \cdot (pO_2 \cdot e^{1.1(PH - 7.2)})^{-1} \cdot 23400) + 1)^{-1}\%$$

Siggaard-Anderson[12]

$$SO_2 = e^{f(PO_2)} \cdot 100/(1 + e^{f(PO_2)})\%$$
$$f/pO_2 \quad = \ln (SO_{20}/(1 - SO_{20})) + \ln (pO_2/pO_{20})$$
$$+ k \cdot \tanh(n_0 - 1) \cdot \ln (pO_2/pO_{20})/k)$$

$SO_{20} \quad = 0.867$

$k \quad = 3.50$

$n_0 \quad = 2.87$

$pO_2 \quad = 1.955 \cdot (P_{50})_{ACT.PH}\ (P_{50})_{7.4} = 26.85$ mm Hg

$(P_{50})_{ACT.PH} = (P_{50})_{7.4} \cdot 10^{-(0.48 \cdot (PH - 7.4))}$

The "gold standard"

The "gold standard" for the calibration of pulse oximetry is the CO-oximeter. The word CO-oximeter was first coined (but not copyrighted) by Instrumentation Laboratories Inc., who released the first commercial CO-oximeter instruments in 1966.

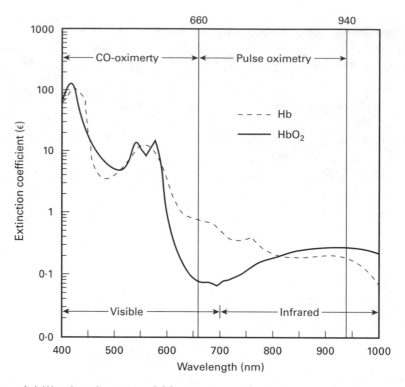

Figure 4.1 Wavelength ranges of CO-oximetry and pulse oximetry.

The CO-oximeter requires small samples of heparinised arterial blood to be taken and, of course, provides oxygen saturation readings only for the instant at which the blood was withdrawn. The CO-oximeter measures the oxygen saturation by a spectrophotometric technique as in pulse oximetry, but none of the commercial devices uses the same wavelengths as current pulse oximeters. Whereas most pulse oximeters use red (660 nm) and near infrared (940 nm), most CO-oximeters operate in the visible range (Figure 4.1), as they work only with haemoglobin solution in plasma, and not with skin, muscle, bone etc. The AVL 912 CO-oximeter is shown in Figure 4.2.

A small (100 µl) heparinised blood sample is introduced into the input port of the CO-oximeter. This sample is haemolysed by ultrasound, and the resulting haemoglobin solution is drawn into a cuvette by a peristaltic pump. As with conventional spectrophotometry, a wideband light source, a tungsten–halogen lamp, is directed through a monochromator. This is a device which reduces the wideband output of the source to a virtually monochromatic—that is, single-coloured—light of very narrow bandwidth. The wavelength of this output is

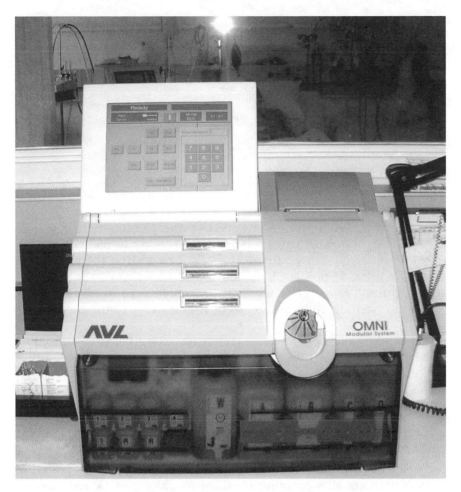

Figure 4.2 AVL 912 CO-oximeter with associated blood gas analyser.

variable over the range 500 nm to 700 nm, controlled by an electric (stepper) motor, so that the light emanating from the monochromator can be scanned. This variable wavelength light is passed through the cuvette containing the haemolysed blood. As the monochromator is controlled by a stepper motor, the wavelength is changed in discrete steps. As this CO-oximeter is designed to measure five components (see Box), only five wavelengths are necessary to make the calculations. However, the sample will contain other absorbents, including fetal haemoglobin, bilirubin, and fragments of the erythrocyte membranes, so the AVL 912 uses up to 17 wavelengths. The light emanating from the cuvette after passing through the blood is detected by a photodiode. The signal from the photodiode is amplified, converted from analogue to digital, and passed to a microprocessor, which makes use of the Beer–Lambert law and simultaneous equations to calculate the values shown in the box.

Values calculated by the CO-oximeter

Measured:	Derived:
Oxyhaemoglobin	Total haemoglobin
Carboxyhaemoglobin	Fractional oxygen saturation
Methaemoglobin	Functional oxygen saturation
"Free" haemoglobin	Oxygen capacity
Sulph haemoglobin	Oxygen content

As so many wavelengths are assessed the AVL CO-oximeter is able to detect many abnormal constituents in the blood sample, which may upset its accuracy. The accuracy is checked by testing the absorption at many different points on the absorption spectra of the expected haemoglobin types. The absorption spectra of many possible abnormal haemoglobins are stored in the software of the machine.

Some CO-oximeters operate using fewer wavelengths. The Radiometer OSM3 Hemoximeter uses six wavelengths. A small sample (35 µl) of heparinised blood is haemolysed in the measurement cuvette by ultrasound at about 40 kHz for a few seconds. This takes place under pressure to stop gases from escaping, and the cuvette is maintained at 37°C. The optical path length is 0·1 mm. Light from a small halogen lamp which has a wide bandwidth of energy is passed through the haemolysed sample, and the light emerging from the cuvette is focused into the monochromator. This spectrum is then applied to a plate with six slits enabling six fixed monochromatic light beams to pass through it. These slits are arranged to allow each of the wavelengths 535 nm, 560 nm, 577 nm, 622 nm, 636 nm and 670 nm to fall on a separate photodiode. The electronic section applies the levels of absorption at each of the six wavelengths to the absorption spectra and calculates the percentages of haemoglobin, oxygenated haemoglobin, carboxyhaemoglobin and methaemoglobin. When fewer wavelengths are used, calibration of the CO-oximeter may be upset by fetal haemoglobin or bilirubin.

Apart from being an *in vitro* rather than an *in vivo* technique, the CO-oximeter differs from the pulse oximeter in the following ways: haemoglobin solution rather than whole blood is used; the optical path length is fixed; there is a different range of wavelengths; the CO-oximeter has more than two wavelengths; and the Beer–Lambert law is more applicable.

In vivo calibration of pulse oximeters

All pulse oximeters developed before 1993 have been calibrated *in vivo*. Because of the methodology of the technique, a multipoint calibration against a CO-oximeter is necessary only during the design and development of the instrument. Once the relation between the oxygen saturation and the absorption ratio of the two wavelengths has been ascertained, a two-point check of calibration is required only for each new combination of light-emitting diode and photodetector. As any deterioration of the light-emitting diodes is likely to be simultaneous or catastrophic and a single photodetector is used, no further calibration checks are usually required. This does not mean that a method of checking the calibration at regular intervals would not be desirable.

In view of the necessity, until now, for *in vivo* calibration, the purchaser and user must understand the problems involved. An indwelling arterial cannula is placed in the radial artery of a fit and healthy volunteer who is a non-smoker and known to have haemoglobin A. Initial blood samples are taken to make sure that the subject's carboxyhaemoglobin and methaemoglobin concentrations are as low as is possible in the healthiest non-smoking population. One or more pulse oximeter probes are placed on the subject's fingers. Initially the subject breathes air, or air with enough added oxygen to raise the arterial saturation to 100%. They then breathe an atmosphere of progressively less oxygen with proportionately more nitrogen. This atmosphere is made progressively more hypoxic by stages, allowing the subject to equilibrate at each new level of arterial oxygen saturation. When the pulse oximeter shows a steady saturation, samples of arterial blood are taken and tested in a CO-oximeter. Thus, by making the subject progressively more hypoxic, a calibration curve of SpO_2 to SaO_2 may be plotted.

Several problems are associated with *in vivo* calibration. First, there is the problem of the ethics of deliberately desaturating a healthy volunteer, even with fully informed consent. Second, it is obvious that one should not deliberately desaturate any subject below about 85% because of the risk of hypoxic brain damage, which may not be apparent at the time. Anecdotal evidence suggests that one such subject in the United States had a convulsion 24 hours after being desaturated at a calibration session. Because of this limitation, it is necessary to extrapolate the calibration curve for values of SpO_2 below 85%. A further problem with *in vivo* calibration is the number and position of the calibration points on the oxyhaemoglobin dissociation curve. If manufacturers of pulse oximeters are asked to disclose how many calibration points are on their curves, they should also disclose their spacing. Having many points clustered between 95% and 100% is far less accurate than having fewer points, well spaced, ranging from 100% down to 80%.

For the calibration to be relevant to all pulse oximeters of a particular model, the light-emitting diodes and photodetectors must be identical in all units that use the calibration curve. As mentioned in Chapter 3, the manufacturer must either carefully select the light-emitting diodes to have their centre wavelengths within close limits, or else measure the centre wavelengths and fit a device to alter calibration in the probe with the diodes. Thus it should be possible to interchange probes, within the limits stated by the manufacturer, without needing to recalibrate the instrument at each change.

The centre wavelength of light-emitting diodes varies with operating current and temperature. The peak wavelength of a diode centred on 660 nm (red) will vary by 5·5 nm with a change of temperature from 0° to 50°C, and a 940 nm (near infrared) diode will vary by 7·8 nm over a similar temperature range. A theoretical computer model based on the Beer–Lambert law showed that over this temperature range a change in the peak wavelength of the diode would cause only a negligible change in the accuracy of the two-wavelength pulse oximeter.[13] Any discrepancy in results obtained *in vivo* is most likely to have been caused by physiological changes in tissue perfusion with change in temperature.

Because of the variation in thickness and pigmentation of the fingers and earlobes on which the pulse oximeter probe is applied, there is a large variation in overall optical density with which the instrument has to cope. In order to keep the AC component of the signal within reasonable limits, most manufacturers arrange for automatic variation of the intensity, usually in steps, until the optimal signal is obtained, within the first few cardiac cycles after application of the probe. The intensity is varied by altering the drive current of the diodes. It has been shown that over the typical range used it may be necessary to alter the diodes' output over the range by a factor of 10. Tests showed that a red diode shifts its peak wavelength by 8 nm over this range, but the shift for the infrared diode is negligible.[14] These results were also applied to a computer model, which showed that if no compensation for this change in wavelength with change in drive current is made then an error of 2·5% would occur at 50% arterial saturation. At saturations of greater than 85%, the model predicts negligible loss of accuracy from this cause.

Accuracy

As mentioned previously, pulse oximeters are calibrated by the use of empirically observed data from several fit adults, and this technique was validated as producing an acceptable accuracy for routine clinical use.[15] Commercial brands vary, however, especially at saturations < 85%.[16] This is because *in vivo* calibration below 80% is unethical, and therefore the calibration curve has to be extrapolated below this value. Most manufacturers specify that their pulse oximeter readings can be expected to have a deviation of 2–3% in the saturation range 70–100%. Almost all units surveyed by many workers fall within this limit.

Mannheimer *et al.*[17] have shown that at high saturations accuracy is best using LEDs of the order of 660 nm and 900 nm, whereas at low saturations 735 nm and 890 nm provide better accuracy.

The accuracy of pulse oximetry may also be affected by haematocrit. Vegfors *et al.*[18] found that reduction of haematocrit from 40% to 11% improved accuracy between SpO_2 86% and 100%, but deteriorated with SpO_2 < 85% in rabbits. Using an *in vitro* model, haemodilution also improved the correlation between SpO_2 and CO-oximetry; there was still further improvement when haemolysis had occurred.[19]

During use, the accuracy of a pulse oximeter on a particular subject may be affected by a number of serious problems, which are described in Chapter 10. In normal use, in patients with only normal adult haemoglobin, HbA, the best accuracy and performance will be attained if the probe is adjusted to attain an arterial signal of the largest amplitude possible; this can be done only if a plethysmograph trace is available.

In vitro calibration

In vitro calibration would be of great advantage in pulse oximetry for the reasons given in the Box.

Several attempts have been made to produce small, inexpensive devices to test the calibration of pulse oximeters without resorting to the use of blood or haemoglobin solutions. However, these *in vitro* test devices suffer from two main disadvantages: only fixed points can be tested with each device; and comparisons between different makes or

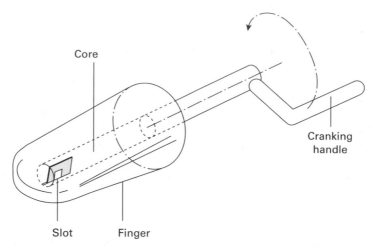

Figure 4.3 Simple test object for assessing pulse oximeters. Reproduced with permission from AJ Munley, MJ Sik, A Shaw. A test object for assessing pulse oximeters. *Lancet* 1989;**i**:1048–9.

Advantages of *in vitro* calibration

- Data points on a calibration curve could extend below 85%
- Calibration studies could be repeated more readily
- No morbidity
- Effects of abnormal haemoglobins may be readily assessed
- Standardisation of calibration possible
- Effects of interfering agents, both physical and chemical, could be tested in a standardised fashion
- Repeated calibration checks by the test houses of the standards organisations and users would be possible

---

models of pulse oximeter are not possible. Nevertheless, simple devices have been developed which may be used as a quick test of pulse oximeter function as long as their limitations are remembered. One such device is shown in Figure 4.3.[20] This consists of a piece of polyester resin cast in the shape of a fingertip. A slot has been cut into the tip and a piece of suitably coloured perspex has been fixed into the slot. Cranking this device in the path of the diodes of a pulse oximeter generates a signal which, for the same make and model of pulse oximeter, produces similar SpO$_2$ values.

Fisher *et al.*[21] describe a simple testing device using dyes to simulate haemoglobin absorption. This is now available commercially from Nonin Medical Inc. Unlike many attempts at non-haemoglobin test devices, this one reportedly shows good correspondence between many different types of pulse oximeter.

The development of a reliable *in vitro* method of calibration which is applicable to a wide range of pulse oximeters is especially important, as several studies have shown increasing inaccuracy as the saturation decreases below 75%, and also increasing differences between the results from different instruments at low saturations.[16,20,22] Several workers in this field have concluded that the versatile *in vitro* calibration systems require circulating blood or haemoglobin solution.[2]

The system developed by Reynolds and colleagues is shown in Figure 4.4. Whole blood that has been anticoagulated with heparin is circulated around a closed loop system by a peristaltic pump. The components of the circuit are a membrane oxygenator, a model finger and a reservoir. A gas-mixing pump supplies a predetermined mixture of oxygen, nitrogen, and small amounts of carbon dioxide to the oxygenator and provides an identical atmosphere at the blood–gas interface in the reservoir. The carbon dioxide is added to maintain the correct pH and PCO_2. A peristaltic pump is used to minimise any damage to the erythrocytes. It is driven by a stepper motor, which is controlled by an IBM-compatible personal computer. With this form of drive system the pulsatile nature of blood flow in the arterial system can be simulated. Two membrane oxygenators were tried. The commercially available Capiox miniature oxygenator works satisfactorily but needs a comparatively large priming volume, 90 ml, of blood. The oxygenator used, developed in Oxford by Dorrington and colleagues, requires only 5 ml of priming blood.[23] It is a parallel plate device, sandwiching a membrane of microporous isotactic polypropylene film. Blood passes one side of the membrane and gases come into contact with the other. The design of the simulated finger is complex, as it has to have the same DC absorption as a human finger and similar diffusion of light, and the AC component of absorption must be similar to that in the physiological state.

To set up the system, a Datex Satlite pulse oximeter was modified so that the red, infrared, AC and DC analogue signals could be displayed on a multichannel oscilloscope. Thus the computer-controlled pump

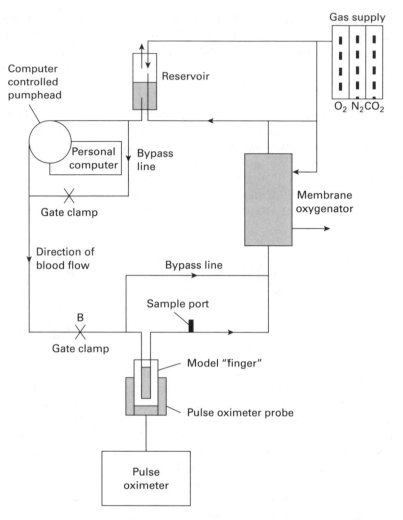

Figure 4.4 *In vitro* test system developed by Reynolds and colleagues.[13]

and the bypass line could be adjusted to simulate physiological conditions in the shape of the waveform, the "heart" rate and the AC:DC ratio. Blood samples were taken from the sample port and tested in a blood gas analyser for correct pH and PCO_2; oxygen saturation as measured by the pulse oximeter under test was measured with a CO-oximeter. Linear regression analysis of the comparison between the Datex Satlite and the CO-oximeter gave an SpO_2 = $0.88SaO_2 + 11.2$ ($r = 0.979$, $p = < 0.001$).

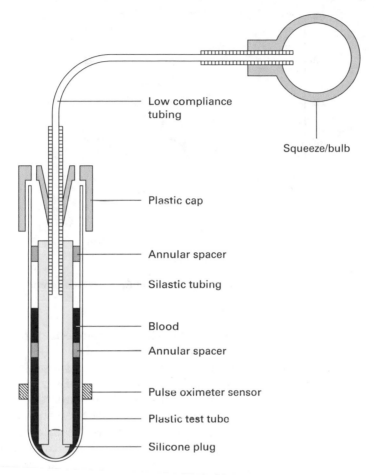

Figure 4.5 Simple device for evaluation of pulse oximetry. Reproduced with permission.[27]

The system has been used to compare 10 commercially available pulse oximeters at saturations of between 50% and 100%, and has been shown to be a valid system for testing the calibration of the technique.[24] As it is a reproducible system, it would be a convenient way of testing the effects of artefacts. The system has also been used to assess the effects of dyshaemoglobins.[25] A similar technique uses a hollow fibre infant oxygenator.[26]

Several devices for *in vitro* evaluations of pulse oximetry have simpler designs. These developments are intended for simple calibration

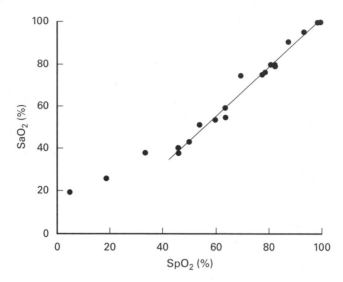

Figure 4.6 Correlation between pulse oximeter and Co-oximeter. Reproduced with permission.[27]

checks by the user or by hospital-based maintenance facilities. One such device, shown in Figure 4.5, requires samples of 0·5–1 ml of blood for each calibration point.[27] It consists of a disposable plastic test tube (12·5 mm × 75 mm) and a 70 mm length of silastic tubing with an inside diameter of 4·4 mm and an outside diameter of 8 mm. The annular space formed between the inside of the test tube and the silastic tubing is deformed at regular intervals by intermittently increasing the air pressure in the silastic tubing by manually squeezing the bulb. Separate samples of heparinised blood are tonometered to different levels of oxygen saturation and each sample is anaerobically tested in turn. The pulse oximeter is applied and the rhythmic squeezing of the bulb is continued until at least 20 seconds of constant amplitude are observed on the plethysmograph tracing. At this point the SpO_2 is recorded and the sample is then transferred anaerobically to a CO-oximeter and the SaO_2 recorded. With this technique an excellent correlation between a Nellcor N100 pulse oximeter and a Radiometer Hemoximeter OSM2b was obtained (Figure 4.6).

Effects of haemoglobin concentration

Theoretically, a wide variation in haemoglobin concentration should make little or no difference to the accuracy of the pulse oximetry technique. With a simple finger model an increasing error was found as haemoglobin concentration deviated from 10 g/dL, SpO_2 being greater than SaO_2 with polycythaemia and less than SaO_2 with anaemia.[27,28] The error increased as the saturation decreased. However, the model used was very simple.

By reducing the packed cell volume in dogs while keeping all other cardiovascular variables as stable as possible by infusions of colloid and crystalloid, the accuracy of both pulse oximetry and continuous mixed venous oxygen saturation was found to be reliable enough for clinical purposes as long as the packed cell volume was > 15%.[29] A slight increase in the scatter at low haematocrit and an underestimation of saturation was also found. When the results of 43 pulse oximeters from 12 manufacturers were pooled the negative bias of the SpO_2 increased approximately linearly from 0 at a haemoglobin concentration of 14 g/dL to −14% at 8 < 9 g/dL at a mean SaO_2 of 53·6%.[30]

The lower limit of haemoglobin *in vivo* at which the pulse oximeter becomes totally unreliable has not yet been determined, as Jay *et al.*[31] have shown good performance as low as 2·3 g/dL.

References

1   Sarnquist FH, Todd C, Whitcher C. Accuracy of a new non-invasive oxygen saturation monitor. *Anesthesiology* 1980;**53**(suppl):S163.
2   Reynolds KJ, Moyle JTB, Gale LB, Sykes MK, Hahn CEW. In vitro performance test system for pulse oximeters. *Med Biol Eng Comput* 1992;**30**:629–35.
3   Van Slyke DD, Neill JM. The determination of gases in the blood and other solutions by vacuum extraction and manometric measurement. *J Biol Chem* 1924;**61**:523–73.
4   Pologe JA. Functional saturation versus fractional saturation: what does the pulse oximeter read. *J Clin Monit* 1989;**5**:298–9.
5   Breuer HWM, Groeben H, Worth H. Oxygen saturation calculation procedures: a critical analysis of six equations for the determination of oxygen saturation. *Intens Care Med* 1989;**15**:385–9.
6   Heck H, Hollmann W. Berechnung der Werte des Säure-Basen-Status mit Hilfe eines Tischcomputers. *Sportarzt Sportmed* 1975;**25**:154.
7   Kelman GR. Digital computer subroutine for the conversion of oxygen tension into saturation. *J Appl Physiol* 1966;**21**.1375.
8   Lutz J, Schulze H-G, Michael UF. Calculation of O_2-saturation and of the oxyhemoglobin dissociation curve for different species, using a new programmable pocket calculator. *Pflügers Arch* 1975;**359**:285.

9 Schulze H-G, Lutz J. Bestimmung von Parametern des Säure-Basen-Haushalts durch programmierbare Taschenrechner. *Med Klin* 1977;**72**: 1429.

10 Marsoner HJ, Harnoncourt K. Berechnung der Sauerstoffsättigung als Funktion von pO_2, pH, Temperatur und Basenabweichung. *Anaesthesist* 1976;**25**:345.

11 Severinghaus JW. Simple, accurate equations for human blood O_2 computations. *J Appl Physiol* 1979;**46**:599.

12 Siggaard-Anderson O. Determination and presentation of acid-base data. *Contrib Nephrol* 1980;**21**:128.

13 Reynolds KJ, de Kock JP, Tarassenko L, Moyle JTB. Temperature dependence of LED and its theoretical effect on pulse oximetry. *Br J Anaesth* 1991;**67**:638–43.

14 De Kock JP, Reynolds KJ, Tarassenko L, Moyle JTB. The effect of varying LED intensity on pulse oximetry. *J Med Eng Technol* 1991;**15**:111–16.

15 Yelderman M, New W. Evaluation of pulse oximetry. *Anesthesiology* 1983; **58**:349–52.

16 Severinghaus JW, Naifeh KH. Accuracy and response of six pulse oximeters to profound hypoxia. *Anesthesiology* 1987;**67**:551–8.

17 Mannheimer PD, Casciani JR, Fein ME, Nierlich SL. Wavelength selection for low-saturation pulse oximetry. *IEEE Trans Biomed Eng* 1997;**44**: 148–58.

18 Vegfors M, Lindberg LG, Oberg PA, Lennmarken C. The accuracy of pulse oximetry at two haematocrit levels. *Acta Anaesthesiol Scand* 1992; **36**:454–9.

19 Vegfors M, Lindberg LG, Oberg PA, Lennmarken C. Accuracy of pulse oximetry at various haematocrits and during haemolysis in an in vitro model. *Med Biol Eng Comput* 1993;**31**:135–41.

20 Munley AJ, Sik MJ, Shaw A. A test object for assessing pulse oximeters. *Lancet* 1989;**i**:1048–9.

21 Fisher JA, Martire T, Volgyesi GA. Evaluation of a new pulse oximeter testing device. *Can J Anaesth* 1996;**43**:179–183.

22 Severinghaus JW, Naifeh KH, Koh SO. Errors in 14 pulse oximeters during profound hypoxia. *J Clin Monit* 1989;**5**:72–81.

23 Dorrington KL, Ralph ME, Bellhouse BJ, Gardaz JP, Sykes MK. Oxygen and CO_2 transfer of a polypropylene dimpled membrane lung with variable secondary flows. *J Biomed Eng* 1985;**7**:90–9.

24 Reynolds KJ, Moyle JTB, Sykes MK, Hahn CEW. Response of 10 pulse oximeters to an in vitro test system. *Br J Anaesth* 1992;**68**:365–9.

25 Reynolds KJ, Palayiwa E, Moyle JTB, Sykes MK, Hahn CEW. The effects of dyshaemoglobins on pulse oximetry. *J Clin Monit* 1993;**9**:81–90.

26 West IP, Griffiths RG, Holmes R, Snowdon SL, Jones GR. In vitro calibration technique for pulse oximeters. Paper given at the 1992 conference of the Association of Anaesthetists.

27 Volgyesi GA, Kolesar R, Lerman J. An in vitro model for evaluating the accuracy of pulse oximeters. *Can J Anaesth* 1990;**37**(suppl):S67.

28 Kolesar R, Volgyesi G, Lerman J. Effect of haemoglobin concentration on the accuracy of pulse oximetry. *Can J Anaesth* 1990;**37**(suppl):S88.
29 Lee SE, Tremper KK, Barker SJ. Effects of anemia on pulse oximetry and continuous mixed venous oxygen saturation monitoring in dogs. *Anesth Analg* 1988;**67**(suppl):S130.
30 Severinghaus JW, Koh SO. Effect of anemia on pulse oximeter accuracy at low saturation. *J Clin Monit* 1990;**6**:85–8.
31 Jay GD, Hughes L, Renzi FP. Pulse oximetry is accurate in acute anemia from hemorrhage. *Ann Emerg Med* 1994;**24**:32–5.

5: Photoplethysmography

Plethysmographic trace

All pulse oximeters should display a plethysmograph trace as well as arterial oxygen saturation and heart rate. The most important function of the plethysmogram in pulse oximetry is to assess whether the pulse oximeter is functioning correctly. The SpO_2 indicated during use should not be relied on unless the plethysmogram bears a strong resemblance to an arterial pressure waveform complete with dicrotic notch (see Figure 2.5, p. 12). The plethysmogram will indicate the presence of mechanical or electrical artefact and whether the pulsatile component of the signal is of sufficient amplitude. However, as will be discussed later, a normal plethysmogram does not necessarily mean that the SpO_2 is correct, as there may be an abnormal haemoglobin or other absorbent circulating. Conventionally, a reduction in transmitted light as occurs in systole leads to an upward deflection of the trace.

During use of the plethysmogram it is vital to know how the software in the pulse oximeter handles the amplitude of the trace. Some manufacturers display the plethysmograph trace "as it comes", whereas others "normalise" the amplitude. The normalised trace is the one presented to the SpO_2 part of the algorithm, but it will not change in amplitude, within certain limits, unless the AC component of the signal becomes too small. Some manufacturers (for example Ohmeda) have a bar graph type of display alongside the plethysmogram, showing the gain applied to the plethysmogram.

Origin of the photoplethysmograph

The photoplethysmograph trace derives from the change of attenuation of the light energy either transmitted or reflected through the tissues over which the pulse oximeter has been applied. This variation in light received by the photodetector depends on the factors indicated in the Box.[1,2]

Comparison between photoplethysmography and strain gauge plethysmography shows a very close correlation ($r = 0.91$ in men,

$r = 0.89$ in women) between the pulsatile component of blood flow in the finger and the change in light absorption.[3] It is possible to separate two main components of the plethysmogram waveform – namely, arterial inflow and venous outflow.[4] If this is possible, then potentially non-invasive information about cardiac function, vascular compliance and peripheral blood flow may be calculated.[5] When the probe is attached to the fingertip or the earlobe, the pulsations detected are almost exclusively from the cutaneous vascular bed.[6] The factors that regulate the blood flow of the skin will have a profound effect on the plethysmogram. An understanding of these factors shows that the information contained in the plethysmogram is of great importance.

Sources of variation in light
- Changes in the amount of blood under the probe
- Erythrocyte orientation
- Erythrocyte concentration
- Rouleau formation
- Local blood velocity
- Separation of light source and detector
- Arterial inflow and venous outflow

The total blood flow of the skin in men may vary from 20 ml/min in the cold to 8 L/min in a hot environment.[7] This is because the main function of cutaneous blood vessels is thermoregulation. Other reflex mechanisms also have an effect on cutaneous blood flow (Figure 5.1). They include baroreceptors, chemoreceptors, humoral mediators both systemic and local, and the higher centre of the brain. Drugs may also act directly on the blood vessels or through the reflex pathways.

To serve the thermoregulatory function the cutaneous vascular bed has many arteriovenous shunts, especially in the extremities. Patency of these shunts increases blood flow and thus heat loss; it also enhances the pulsatility of the venules and small veins, which increases the amplitude of the AC portion of the plethysmogram.[8] Arteriovenous shunts are especially common in the fingers, and therefore the cutaneous vessels of the fingers are more responsive to vasoactive control than are vessels in other areas.

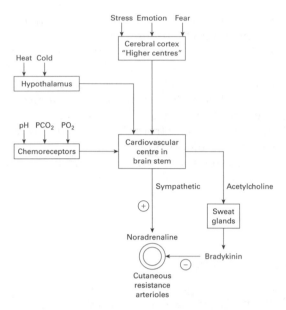

Figure 5.1 Effect of reflex mechanisms on cutaneous blood flow.

Factors affecting cutaneous blood flow

Neurogenic factors
   Sympathetic vasoconstrictor fibres (arterioles, venules, arteriovenous shunts)
   Cholinergic pathway to sweat glands (cause vasodilation)
Reflex vasoconstriction in skin
   Local or central cooling
   Hypotension
   Painful stimuli
   Fear
   Deep inspiration
Reflex vasodilatation in the skin
   Heating (local or general)
   Stimulation of chemoreceptor
   Coronary occlusion
   (Acute hypertension)
Humoral control of cutaneous vasculature
   α-Adrenergic (vasoconstriction)
   Serotonin (vasoconstriction)
   Prostaglandin $F_{2\alpha}$ (vasoconstriction)
   (Vasopressin – vasoconstriction)
   (Angiotensin – vasoconstriction)
Other factors
   Systemic hypoxaemia or hypercapnia (reflex reduction in blood flow to hand)
   Hypercapnia (local effect in vasodilatation)
   Autoregulation (minor role)

Many drugs that affect the autonomic nervous system either directly or as a side effect may affect the cutaneous blood flow and hence the photoplethysmogram. During anaesthesia and intensive care, changes caused by disease or drugs are likely to be observed only if they cause changes during observation. Halothane, nitrous oxide, diethyl ether, isoflurane and thiopentone all cause vasodilatation in the cutaneous vasculature of the finger,[7] but the effects of these factors on the plethysmogram are also influenced by changes in cardiac output.

Assessment of cardiac rhythm

The plethysmogram gives a quick indication of the cardiac rhythm and any change in its regularity. It also shows any compromise in diastolic refilling in bigeminy or with other ectopic rhythms. Sudden changes in cardiac output or hypovolaemia will be indicated by a decreased amplitude in the trace, but this will happen only when the plethysmogram reflects the pulse volume without "normalisation". Hypovolaemia may also be indicated by rhythmic change in the amplitude in synchronism with the phase of the respiration.[9] This is similar to the effect with intra-arterial pressure monitoring, in that the amplitude of the peaks of the pulse waveform show an increased variation in response to positive-pressure ventilation when a patient becomes hypovolaemic.

Assessment of systolic blood pressure

If a sphygmomanometer cuff is applied to the same limb as the pulse oximeter probe, the plethysmogram may be used to assess systolic blood pressure: allow the inflated cuff to deflate, and note the pressure at which the trace just reappears. This correlates well with a similar technique that uses Doppler ultrasound to detect blood flow under the cuff.[10]

Comparing systolic blood pressure measured with a pulse oximeter with blood pressure measured with two other methods – namely Korotkoff sounds and the non-invasive automatic blood pressure monitor utilising the oscillometric principle – Chawla *et al.* found good correlation in 100 healthy volunteers.[11] They also concluded that this was the ideal method of measuring systolic pressure in Takayasu's syndrome (pulseless disease), where conventional techniques often fail.

Allen's test (to assess the patency of the palmar arterial arch) is much simplified by applying the pulse oximeter to the first finger and noting the effect of compression of the radial artery.

Assessment of vascular tone

Continuous monitoring of changes in peripheral vascular resistance may be a possibility in the near future. Shelly *et al.*[12] compared the photoplethysmograph waveform generated by pulse oximetry with the waveform from a direct arterial pressure monitoring system. The qualitative changes in "compliance" (volume change per unit pressure change) were calculated. Vasoconstrictors noradrenaline (norepinephrine) and adrenaline (epinephrine) were shown to decrease compliance as predicted. The results of a case study were sufficient to generate a dose–response curve. This may become a very valuable tool in the management of the critically ill.

Finger or ear?

Photoplethysmograms recorded simultaneously from the finger and the pinna of the ear differ appreciably.[13] Changes in pulse pressure during induction, maintenance of and recovery from anaesthesia are greater when recorded from the finger than from the ear. The plethysmogram should therefore be recorded from the finger whenever possible, to gain the greatest amount of clinically useful information.

Waveforms

If the photoplethysmograph trace is completely unprocessed, the recording may be seen to be comprised of two waveforms, an arterial waveform superimposed on a slower respiratory waveform. The amplitude of the respiratory waveform depends on central venous pressure and intrathoracic pressure.[14] During intermittent positive-pressure ventilation the amplitude is inversely related to central venous pressure.[15]

Other considerations

Disappearance of the plethysmograph trace during anaesthesia should always be investigated immediately. The commonest cause is displacement of the probe, but may be due to cardiac arrest or compression of an end artery causing peripheral ischaemia. It may be possible to use the pulse oximeter to assess the adequacy of external cardiac massage, but any trace is more likely to be due to mechanical artefact, and any SpO_2 value indicated should be treated with suspicion.

An important, if rare, use of the pulse oximeter plethysmogram is to monitor the integrity of the circulation of reimplanted limbs and fingers. Also, a sterile probe could be used to assess the perfusion of, for example, the intestines at operation.

References

1   Weinman J, Hayat A, Raviv G. Reflection photoplethysmography of arterial blood-volume pulses. *Med Biol Eng Comput* 1977;**15**:22–31.
2   Roberts VC. Photoplethysmography – fundamental aspects of the optical properties of blood in motion. *Trans IMC* **4**:101–6.
3   De Trafford J, Lafferty K. What does photoplethysmography measure? *Med Biol Eng Comput* 1984;**22**:479–80.
4   Cook LB. Extracting arterial flow waveforms from pulse oximeter waveforms. *Anaesthesia* 2001;**56**:551–5.
5   Wisely NA, Cook LB. Arterial flow waveforms from pulse oximetry compared with measured Doppler flow waveforms. *Anaesthesia* 2001;**56**:556–61.
6   Hertzman AB. The blood supply to various skin areas as estimated by the photoelectric plethysmograph. *Am J Physiol* 1938;**124**:328.
7   Heistad DD, Abboud FM. Factors that influence blood flow in skeletal muscle and skin. *Anesthesiology* 1974;**41**:139–56.
8   Kim J-M, Arakawa K, Benson KT, Fox DK. Pulse oximetry and circulatory kinetics associated with pulse volume amplitude measured by photoelectric plethysmography. *Anesth Analg* 1986;**65**:1333–9.
9   Partridge BL. Use of pulse oximetry as a non-invasive indicator of intravascular volume status. *J Clin Monit* 1987;**3**:263–8.
10 Korbon GA, Wills MH, D'Lauro F, Lawson D. Systolic blood pressure measurement: Doppler vs pulse-oximeter [abstract]. *Anaesthesiology* 1987;**67**:A188.
11 Chawla R, Kumarval V, Girdhar KK, Sethi AK, Indryan A, Bhattacharya A. Can pulse oximetry be used to measure systolic blood pressure? *Anesth Analg* 1992;**74**:196–200.
12 Shelly KH, Marray WB, Chang D. Arterial-pulse oximetry loops: a new method of monitoring vascular tone. *J Clin Monit* 1997;**13**:223–8.
13 Nijboer JA, Dorlas JC. Comparison of plethysmograms taken from finger and pinna during anaesthesia. *Br J Anaesth* 1985;**57**:531–4.

14 Dorlas JC, Nijboer JA. Photoelectric plethysmography as a monitoring device in anaesthesia: application and interpretation. *Br J Anaesth* 1985;57:524–30.
15 Partridge BL, Sanford TJ. Finger plethysmography in anesthesia. *Semin Anesth* 1989;8:102–11.

6: Physiology of oxygen transport

Since the 1960s, when the blood gas analyser became a routine instrument, most clinicians have thought in terms of the partial pressure of oxygen carried in the blood; oxygen saturation was considered only by the cardiologist in the catheter laboratory and by intensivists when calculating oxygen flux. Oxygen saturation is, in fact, a much more useful concept than partial pressure if the patient has normal adult haemoglobin, as it is only one step away from knowing how much oxygen, by volume, is being transported by the blood – the oxygen flux (see Box). This ignores the volume of oxygen in solution in the plasma, as this is a very small amount compared to that carried by the haemoglobin, for a man breathing air at normal barometric pressure.

> Oxygen flux = cardiac output × arterial oxygen saturation × haemoglobin concentration × 1·39 (where 1·39 is ml of oxygen carried by 1 g of haemoglobin)

Oxyhaemoglobin dissociation curve

It is important to understand the relationship between the partial pressure of oxygen in the plasma and the affinity and hence the saturation of the haemoglobin molecule with oxygen. The affinity of oxygen to haemoglobin may be shown by the oxyhaemoglobin dissociation curve (Figure 6.1); it is also important to understand the factors that affect the position of the curve.

A complete oxyhaemoglobin dissociation curve can be plotted automatically. One apparatus for doing this is the Hemox-Analyser (TCS Medical Products, Huntingdon Valley, Pennsylvania). This device (Figure 6.2) measures oxygen saturation spectrophotometrically while measuring the partial pressure oxygen in the cuvette that contains the sample of blood. The partial pressure of the oxygen is varied automatically from zero to a pressure that results in full saturation in

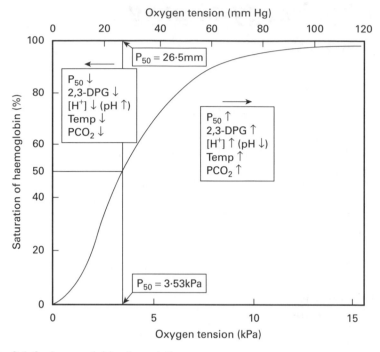

Figure 6.1 Oxyhaemoglobin dissociation curve.

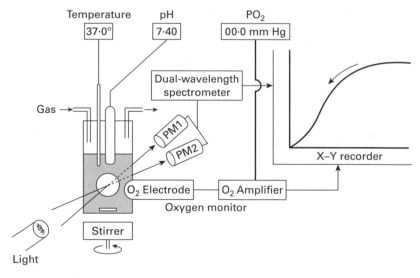

Figure 6.2 To plot the oxyhaemoglobin dissociation curve automatically, the Hemox-Analyser simultaneously measures oxygen saturation and the partial pressure of oxygen from a blood sample. Reproduced courtesy of TCS Medical Products Co.

about 10 minutes. Only two wavelengths are used, and therefore the apparatus is calibrated only for specific known haemoglobins.

Position of the curve

As the curve, in the main, shifts to the left or right in a parallel fashion, its actual position is often denoted by the P_{50}, which is the partial pressure of oxygen when the haemoglobin is 50% saturated at a plasma pH of 7·4 and a temperature of 37°C. The normal value of P_{50} is approximately 3·5 kPa. The effects of a shift in the curve are shown in the Box.

Effects of a shift in the oxyhaemoglobin dissociation curve

Shift to the left	*Shift to the right*
Increased affinity	Decreased affinity
Decreased P_{50}	Increased P_{50}
Impaired oxygenation	Facilitation of oxygenation

The sigmoid shape of the oxyhaemoglobin dissociation curve has physiological advantages. The flat upper part means that the oxygen loading in the lungs is little affected by small changes in the partial pressure of the oxygen with which the blood comes into contact. Also, as the erythrocyte takes up oxygen as it passes along the length of the pulmonary capillary, a large partial pressure difference between the alveolar gas and the blood persists even when most of the oxygen has been transferred from the gas phase. This results in the process being speeded up. When the blood reaches the peripheral tissues, the steep lower part of the curve allows rapid transfer of large amounts of oxygen from the haemoglobin to the tissues for only a small drop in capillary oxygen tension.[1]

The causes of the displacement of the oxyhaemoglobin dissociation curve are summarised in the Box on p. 62. In 1904 Bohr elucidated the effect that bears his name: the shift of the oxyhaemoglobin dissociation curve due to changes in hydrogen ion concentration (Figure 6.3). The clinical significance of the Bohr effect is that a shift of the curve to the right aids the release of oxygen at tissue level but impairs the oxygenation of haemoglobin in the lungs. The oxyhaemoglobin dissociation curve is also shifted by changes in the partial pressure of carbon dioxide (Figure 6.4) and in temperature (Figure 6.5).

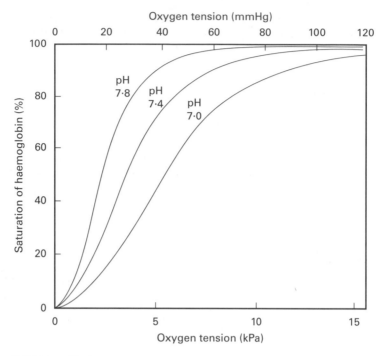

Figure 6.3 Bohr effect.

Certain abnormal haemoglobins have shifted oxyhaemoglobin dissociation curves. $Hb_{Chesapeake}(P_{50} = 19$ mmHg$)$ and $Hb_{SanDiego}$ $(P_{50} = 16·4$ mmHg$)$ have an increased oxygen affinity, whereas $Hb_{Kansas}(P_{50} = 70$ mmHg$)$ has a reduced oxygen affinity.[2]

Causes of displacement of the oxyhaemoglobin curve

Left displacement
Decrease in hydrogen ion concentration (increase in pH)
Decrease in temperature
Decrease in PCO_2
Decrease in 2,3-DPG in red blood cells
Decrease in ATP in red blood cells
Increase in carboxyhaemoglobin
Increase in methaemoglobin
Abnormal haemoglobins

Right displacement
Increase in hydrogen ion concentration (decrease in pH)
Increase in temperature
Increase in PCO_2
Increase in 2,3-DPG in red blood cells
Increase in ATP in red blood cells
Decrease in zinc in red blood cells
Abnormal haemoglobins

All phosphates exert an effect on oxygen affinity and hence the position of the oxyhaemoglobin dissociation curve. Chanutin and

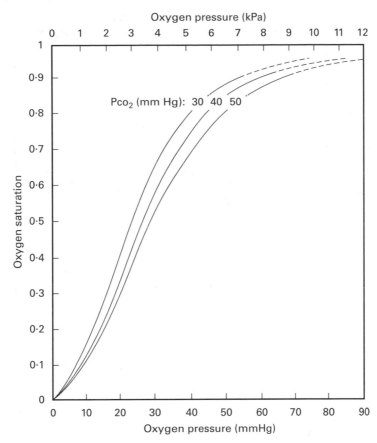

Figure 6.4 Shift in oxyhaemoglobin dissociation curve with change in partial pressure of carbon dioxide.

Curnish showed that 2,3-disphosphoglycerate (2,3-DPG) and adenosine triphosphate (ATP) were the only phosphates of significant concentration in the red blood cell.[3] 2,3-DPG has a considerable controlling effect on the oxygen affinity of haemoglobin. An increase in erythrocyte 2,3-DPG concentration reduces the affinity of haemoglobin for oxygen, and vice versa. Therefore, an increase in 2,3-DPG concentration improves tissue oxygenation, whereas a decrease may lead to tissue hypoxia.[4] This tissue hypoxia may of course occur despite normal or high values of indicated arterial oxygen saturation from a pulse oximeter or partial pressure as measured with a blood gas analyser.

The outline of the metabolism of 2,3-DPG is shown in Figure 6.6. The Embden–Myerhof anaerobic pathway is the predominant

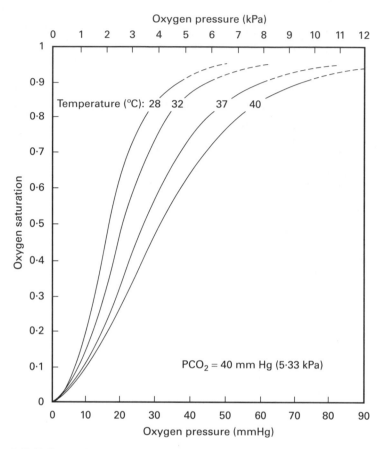

Figure 6.5 Shift in oxyhaemoglobin dissociation curve with change in temperature.

method of metabolism of glucose in the red blood cell. About a fifth of the glucose metabolised in this pathway passes down a shunt. It should be noted also that another important shunt associated with the Embden–Myerhof pathways is that of methaemoglobin reductase. The methaemoglobin reductase shunt maintains the reduced state of the iron in the haem. This is further discussed in Chapter 11.

The concentration of 2,3-DPG in the red cell is normally controlled by a negative feedback mechanism from 2,3-DPG itself. Other factors causing variation in 2,3-DPG concentration are shown in the Box on p. 66.

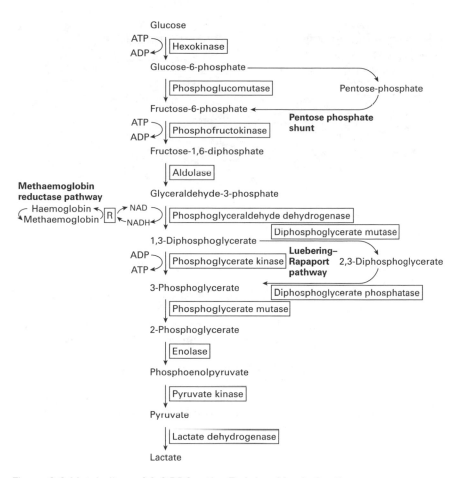

Figure 6.6 Metabolism of 2,3-DPG – the Embden–Myerhof pathway.

Stored blood suffers a steady decline in its 2,3-DPG concentration. All the 2,3-DPG is depleted within three weeks, with acid–citrate–dextrose preservative causing a fall in P_{50} to approximately 2 kPa (15 mmHg). When citrate–phosphate–dextrose is used as the preservative the depletion rate is much slower.[5] If large amounts of blood that has been stored to the limit of its viability are transfused, then the overall change in P_{50} for the patient will shift to the left, but usually only by about 0·5 kPa (3·8 mmHg). The concentration of 2,3-DPG in the transfused erythrocytes will return to normal values in three or four hours.

Causes of fluctuation in 2,3-DPG concentration in erythrocytes

Decrease in 2,3-DPG
    Increased hydrogen ion concentration
    Hexokinase deficiency
    Hypophosphataemia
    Hyperthyroidism
    Old erythrocytes
    Stored blood

Increase in 2,3-DPG
    Decreased hydrogen ion concentration
    Pyruvate kinase deficiency
    Hyperphosphataemia
    Hypothyroidism
    Young erythrocytes
    Anaemia
    ?Altitude

References

1 West JB. *Respiratory physiology – the essentials*. Baltimore: Williams & Wilkins, 1990.
2 Bellingham AJ. Haemoglobins with altered oxygen affinity. *Br Med Bull* 1976;**32**:234–8.
3 Chanutin A, Curnish RR. Effect of organic and inorganic phosphates on the oxygen equilibrium of human erythrocytes. *Biochem Biophys* 1967; **121**:96.
4 MacDonald R. Red cell 2,3-diphosphoglycerate and oxygen affinity. *Anaesthesia* 1977;**32**:544–53.
5 Shafer AW, Tague LL, Welch MH, Guenter CA. 2,3-Diphosphoglycerate in red cells stored in acid-citrate-dextrose and citrate-phosphate-dextrose. *J Lab Clin Med* 1971;**77**:430.

7: Pulse oximetry at high altitude

There is no theoretical or engineering reason for the technique of pulse oximetry to be inaccurate at high altitude. In the case of high altitude *and* low ambient temperature, failure may be due to poor peripheral perfusion.

In discussing the use of pulse oximetry at high altitude there are two distinct situations, namely sudden changes in altitude, as in flying in aircraft, and changes that occur slowly with acclimatisation, or even *very* slowly in the case of those living at high altitude.

The general term for inhalation of an atmosphere which has a low partial pressure of oxygen due to increased altitude is *hypobaric hypoxia*, that is, the *fractional* proportion of oxygen remains 0·21 but the ambient barometric pressure is reduced.

Effects of high altitude

Atmospheric pressure falls with increasing altitude; as the pressure falls the partial pressure of oxygen also falls, despite the concentration remaining constant. As a consequence of the drop in PiO_2 there is a fall in P_AO_2 and hence oxygen saturation. To a certain extent the fall in P_AO_2 is less than the fall in PiO_2 as there is a concomitant fall in P_ACO_2 due to hyperventilation. There is a shift to the right in the oxyhaemoglobin dissociation curve caused by an increase in 2,3-DPG, which in turn is caused by hypoxia. This shift is counteracted by an opposite shift caused by the decrease in PCO_2. Therefore, the "normal" SpO_2 for a given altitude can only be approximate (Figure 7.1).

When estimating the inspired PO_2 it must be remembered that as altitude increases and barometric pressure falls, fractional concentration and the saturated vapour pressure (SVP) of water at body temperature remain constant. Therefore:

Table 7.1 Barometric pressure relative to altitude

Altitude		Barometric pressure		Inspired gas PO$_2$		Equivalent oxygen per cent at sea level	Percentage oxygen required to give sea level value of inspired gas PO$_2$
feet	metres	kPa	mmHg	kPa	mmHg		
0	0	101	760	19.9	149	20.9	20.9
2 000	610	94.3	707	18.4	138	19.4	22.6
4 000	1 220	87.8	659	16.9	127	17.8	24.5
6 000	1 830	81.2	609	15.7	118	16.6	26.5
8 000	2 440	75.2	564	14.4	108	15.1	28.8
10 000	3 050	69.7	523	13.3	100	14.0	31.3
12 000	3 660	64.4	483	12.1	91	12.8	34.2
14 000	4 270	59.5	446	11.1	83	11.6	37.3
16 000	4 880	54.9	412	10.1	76	10.7	40.8
18 000	5 490	50.5	379	9.2	69	9.7	44.8
20 000	6 100	46.5	349	8.4	63	8.8	49.3
22 000	6 710	42.8	321	7.6	57	8.0	54.3
24 000	7 320	39.2	294	6.9	52	7.3	60.3
26 000	7 930	36.0	270	6.3	47	6.6	66.8
28 000	8 540	32.9	247	5.6	42	5.9	74.5
30 000	9 150	30.1	226	4.9	37	5.2	83.2
35 000	10 700	23.7	178	3.7	27	3.8	–
40 000	12 200	18.8	141	2.7	20	2.8	–
45 000	13 700	14.8	111	1.8	13	1.9	–
50 000	15 300	11.6	87	1.1	8	1.1	–
63 000	19 200	6.3	47	0	0	0	–

100% oxygen restores sea level inspired PO$_2$ at 10 000 metres (33 000 ft). Reproduced with permission[1].

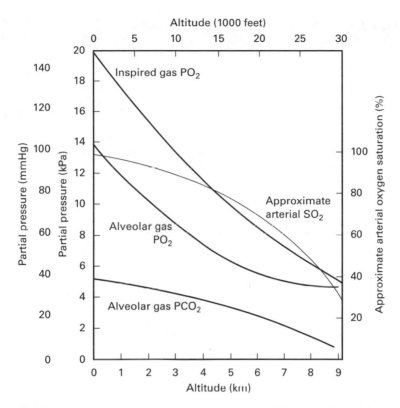

Figure 7.1 Approximate arterial oxygen saturation as a function of altitude.

Inspired $PO_2 = 0.21$(barometric pressure $- 6.3$) kPa

Inspired $PO_2 = 0.21$(barometric pressure $- 47$) mmHg

The significance of SVP increases is altitude. At approximately 19 000 metres (63 000 ft) the barometric pressure equals the water vapour pressure, the body fluids boil and alveolar PO_2 and PCO_2 fall to zero.[1]

The susceptibility to the effects of high altitude on individuals depends on a number of factors:[2]

• The intensity of the hypoxia

    − maximum altitude attained
    − duration
    − rate of ascent
    − rate of descent

Table 7.2 *Approximate* symptomatology of exposure to high altitude

Altitude	Acute	Full acclimatisation
29 000 feet	LOC within 2–3 minutes	Limit of climbing without supplementary oxygen
20 000 feet	LOC within 10 minutes	Limit of continuous climbing without supplementary oxygen. Highest permanent habitation
12 000–20 000 feet	Amnesia, dizziness, breathless at rest	Breathless on exertion
10 000–12 000 feet	Insomnia Anorexia	
8 000–10 000 feet	Breathless on exertion Impaired night vision	

- Physical activity
    - exercise exacerbates symptoms/signs
- Ambient temperature
    - cold environment reduces tolerance to hypoxia
- Intercurrent illness
- Ingestion of certain drugs, including alcohol
    - e.g. antihistamines.

The symptomatology of acute and chronic exposure to altitude is shown in Table 7.2.

Acclimatisation

There is a wide variation in the ability of an individual to cope with high altitude, depending on "acclimatisation", which occurs over periods of days to months depending on the altitudes it is necessary to attain.

- Increase in CSF carbonic anhydrase activity to correct shift in CSF pH due to lower $PaCO_2$
- Polycythaemia to increase oxygen carriage
- Increase in 2,3-DPG to increase oxygen delivery to the tissues at a lower PaO_2
- Reduced vascular response to hypoxia (reduces risk of high-altitude pulmonary oedema, HAPE).

In the well acclimatised it may be difficult to know what the "normal" SpO_2 should be. In the neonate born at 1610 m (5280 ft),

Thilo *et al.*[3] found that 24 hours after birth the mean SpO_2 of a group of 150 healthy babies was 92–93%, increasing to 93–94% in the awake state. This fell to as low as 85% during feeding. At 1–3 months of age SpO_2 fell to as low as 86% during sleep and 88–89% during activity.

Nicholas *et al.*[4] found the mean SpO_2 of healthy infants living at 2800 m (9000 ft) to be 91·7%. It appears that in those native to high altitude, oxygen saturation increases from infancy to childhood and then decreases during adulthood.[5]

Reuland *et al.*[6] and Lozano *et al.*[7] have shown that pulse oximetry is a good objective diagnostic tool in children living in small communities at high altitude where radiology is not available. There is even a significant fall in SpO_2 in children with mild upper respiratory tract infection at moderate altitude (1500 m).[8]

Flying at high altitude

The situation with hypoxia and flying is very different from living at high altitude, as there is no acclimatisation. Two situations need to be considered: the effects of commercial aviation, and the intentional or unintentional exposure to very high altitudes. Air travel is now universally in "pressurised" aircraft. It is often assumed that aircraft are pressurised to the atmospheric pressure at sea level, but this is not the case: the majority of commercial aircraft cabins are pressurised to the equivalent of 8000 feet above sea level. This is referred to as *cabin altitude*. The reason for this is that if the cabin were pressurised to sea level pressure the structure of the aircraft would have to be significantly stronger to withstand the differential pressure of flying at high altitude. There would also be a large fuel penalty, as the aircraft would be heavier and more energy would be required to maintain the higher cabin pressure. Although 8000 ft cabin altitude may seem reasonable, one must remember that approximately half the air in the cabin is recirculated through the air conditioning system (known in the industry as "air con packs"). This means that the fractional amount of oxygen is lower than 0·21, and the level of carbon dioxide is allowed to rise to 3% in older aircraft and 0·5% in newer aircraft. Also, at the very high altitude at which most airliners fly, the air that is pumped into the cabin is very dry because the outside cabin air humidity is often < 10%. It is too expensive for the aircraft manufacturers to rehumidify the air in the cabin. Further, even on the most modern aircraft the methods of controlling the cabin altitude are relatively crude. Surprisingly, the partial pressure of oxygen in the cabin

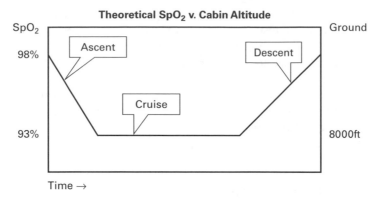

Figure 7.2 Variance in SpO$_2$ during commercial flight.

atmosphere is not monitored. This is because physiologists are not involved in aircraft design: the physiology used is based on experiments done during the second world war. There is a lack of understanding that the human body requires a minimum *partial pressure* of oxygen, rather than ambient overall atmospheric pressure.

It is also surprising that with the advent of pulse oximetry there have not been many investigations into what is actually occurring as far as oxygenation is concerned in commercial flight. Figure 7.2 shows theoretically how SpO$_2$ should change during a flight.

A key paper by Cottrell *et al.*[9] shows that all is not what it should be. Using pulse oximetry, the arterial oxygen saturation of 42 airline crew members was continuously monitored on 22 scheduled flights. Mean nadir arterial oxygen saturation fell from 97% pre-flight to 88·6% at cruising altitudes. The results revealed large variations between individuals. Individual nadir saturations ranged from 93% down to 80%, and it must be remembered that these results are from healthy aircrew. Figure 7.3 shows one subject's SpO$_2$ during one flight. Figure 7.4 is a plot of cabin altitude versus minimum SpO$_2$ for the 42 crew members tested.

The variations from the expected SpO$_2$ may have been due to:

- Inaccuracy in the cabin altitude controller
- Age (29–59 years)
- Smokers (5·3% current but 23% ex-smokers)
- Medications (16%)
- General health
- Length of flight
- Time of flight (awake/asleep).

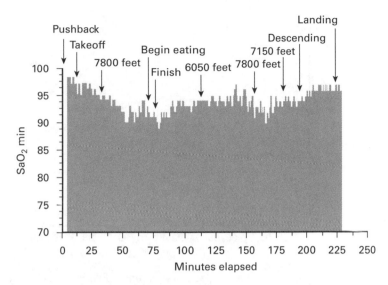

Figure 7.3 Graph of one subject's saturation over one flight. Values given represent recorded cabin altitudes.

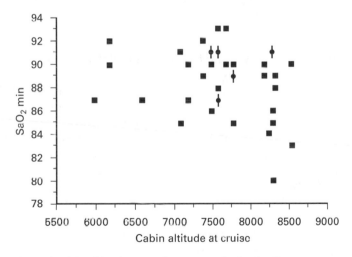

Figure 7.4 Plot of cabin altitude at cruise versus SaO_2min. Squares represent one crew member. Squares with lines indicate two crew members.

Nevertheless, if this is what happens with reasonably fit aircrew, it should be of great concern what occurs with the random air passenger. Ernsting,[10] for several decades the leading flight physiologist, advocated the reduction of cabin altitude from a maximum of 8000 ft to a maximum of 6000 ft, but to no avail.

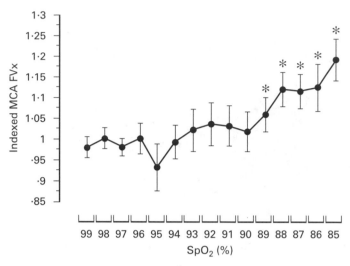

Figure 7.5 Effect of gradual stepwise desaturation on middle cerebral artery maximal flow velocity (MCA FVx) measured using transcranial Doppler. All values for each subject are indexed to the initial value obtained. *Values (mean ± 95% confidence interval) of middle cerebral artery maximal flow velocity are significantly different from baseline ($p < 0.05$).

Concern over the effect of mild hypoxia in flight deck personnel should have been heightened by some work done in Cambridge (UK) published in 1997 by Gupta *et al*.[11] Unrelated to flying, this team investigated, non-invasively, the effects of hypoxaemia on cerebral vasculature. Thirteen healthy volunteers were studied using transcranial Doppler sonography. Time-averaged middle cerebral artery maximal flow velocity (MCA FVx), mean arterial blood pressure, peripheral oxygen saturation (SpO_2), and partial pressure of end-tidal CO_2 were measured at baseline and during a graded reduction in arterial SpO_2 to 85%, at normocapnia. Flow velocity and estimated cerebrovascular resistance (CVR_e) were indexed and plotted against SpO_2. As is shown in the plots in Figures 7.5 and 7.6 there is a sudden and statistically significant cerebral vasodilatation when SpO_2 decreases below 90%. The questions that must be asked in relation to flying are:

- Is this the brain showing distress at lack of oxygen?
- Is there likely to be a sudden reduction in the efficiency of cognition, with concomitant increased risk of human error on the flight deck?
- Could this be one of the triggers in the cause of disruptive passenger behaviour or "air rage"?

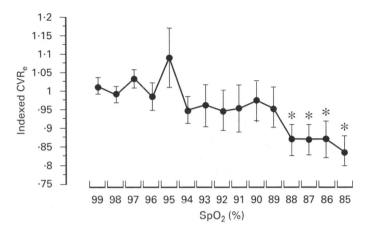

Figure 7.6 Effect of gradual stepwise desaturation on indexed cerebrovascular resistance (CVR_e) measured using transcranial Doppler and continuous plethysmographic blood pressure. All values for each subject are indexed to the initial value obtained. *Values (mean ± 95% confidence interval) of cerebrovascular resistance are significantly different from baseline ($p < 0.05$).

Fitness for flight

A common question posed to physicians is "is this individual fit to fly as a passenger?" This is a more important question than many realise, as patients who are normally mildly hypoxic due, for example, to COPD, may suddenly decompensate at a cabin cruise altitude of 8000 ft with severe hypoxia occurring secondary to HAPE. The question of fitness to fly can only be answered here from the point of view of tests for oxygenation. Ideally, the patient should be subjected to a trial in a hypobaric chamber. Unfortunately, this equipment is expensive, rare, and not available at district general hospitals, but a simple test has been developed by Robson et al.[12] in Edinburgh. A hypoxia inhalation test (HIT) is conducted. Baseline oxygen saturation (SpO_2) is measured using a pulse oximeter. If SpO_2 is < 90% no HIT is performed and the patient is assessed as unfit for air travel. If the baseline SpO_2 is ≥ 90% an HIT is performed by the patient breathing through a 35% Venturi mask supplied with 100% nitrogen, which reduces the inspiratory fraction to 15·1+/–0·2%. The algorithm used to decide whether the subject is fit to fly is shown in Figure 7.7.

A good review of altitude-related pulmonary disorders has been published by Krieger and de la Hoz.[13]

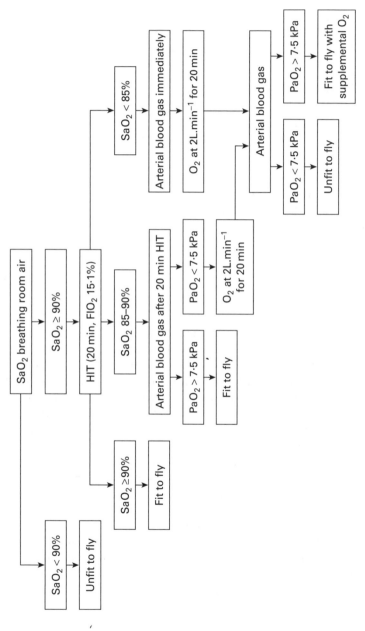

Figure 7.7 Baseline arterial oxygen saturation (SaO_2) was measured whilst breathing air for 5 min. HIT: hypoxia inhalation test; FIO_2: inspiratory oxygen fraction; PaO_2: arterial oxygen pressure; A: fit to fly; B: fit to fly with supplemental oxygen; C: unfit to fly. Reproduced with permission[12].

References

1 Nunn J. *Applied respiratory physiology*. Oxford: Butterworth–Heinemann, 1999.

2 Harding RM revised by Gradwell DR. Hypoxia and hyperventilation. In: Ernstine J *et al. Aviation medicine*, 3rd edn. Oxford: Edward Arnold, 1999.

3 Thilo EH, Park-Moore B, Berman ER, Carson BS. Oxygen saturation by pulse oximetry in healthy infants at an altitude of 1610 m (5280 ft). What is normal? *Am J Dis Child* 1991;**145**:1137–40.

4 Nicholas R, Yaron M, Reeves J. Oxygen saturation in children living at moderate altitude. *J Am Fam Pract* 1993;**6**:452–6.

5 Beall CM. Oxygen saturation increases during childhood and decreases during adulthood among high altitude native Tibetians residing at 3800–4000 m. *High Alt Med Biol* 2000;**1**:25–32.

6 Reuland DS, Steinhoff MC, Gilman RH *et al*. Prevalence and prediction of hypoxemia in children with respiratory infections in the Peruvian Andes. *J Pediatr* 1991;**119**:900–6.

7 Lozano JM, Steinhoff M, Ruiz JG, Mesa ML, Martinez N. Clinical predictors of acute radiological pneumonia and hypoxaemia at high altitude. *Arch Dis Child* 1994;**71**:323–7.

8 Beebe SA, Heery LB, Magarian S, Culberson J. Pulse oximetry at moderate altitude. Healthy children and children with upper respiratory infection. *Clin Pediatr* 1994;**33**:329–32.

9 Cottrell JJ, Lebovitz BL, Fennell RG, Kohn GM. Inflight arterial saturation: continuous monitoring by pulse oximetry. *Space Environ Med* 1995;**66**:126–30.

10 Ernsting J. The 10th Annual Harry G Armstrong Lecture: Prevention of hypoxia – acceptable compromises. *Aviat Space Environ Med* 1978;**49**:495–502.

11 Gupta AK, Menon DK, Czosnyka M, Smielewski P, Jones JG. Thresholds for hypoxic cerebral vasodilation in volunteers. *Anesth Analg* 1997;**85**:817–20.

12 Robson AG, Hartung TK, Innes JA. Laboratory assessment of fitness to fly in patients with lung disease: a practical approach. *Eur Respir J* 2000;**16**:214–9.

13 Krieger B, de la Hoz RE. Altitude-related pulmonary disorders. *Crit Care Clin* 1999;**15**:265–80.

8: General clinical applications

The clinical applications of pulse oximetry in medicine are as important as oxygen is to life. This may seem an overstatement, but as more and more pulse oximeters are coming into use, an increasing number of hypoxaemic events are being seen as precursors of pathological events. This chapter gives an overview of the applications of pulse oximetry. It is followed by chapters on special areas of importance and on the clinical limitations of the technique.

The applications of photoplethysmography, assuming that the pulse oximeter in use displays such a trace, have been discussed in Chapter 5. All pulse oximeters should display a plethysmogram, as one of the functions of such a display is to help verify the indicated oxyhaemoglobin saturation value.

Oxygen lack

In 1921 JS Haldane said: "Oxygen lack not only stops the machine but wrecks the machinery". Oxygen lack at the cellular level may be categorised into one of four types (Box).

Types of oxygen lack at cellular level
- Hypoxic hypoxia – arterial haemoglobin oxygen saturation is low
- Anaemic hypoxia – the haemoglobin may be fully saturated with oxygen but haemoglobin concentration is too low
- Stagnant hypoxia – either cardiac output is too low or there is complete vessel occlusion
- Histotoxic or cytotoxic hypoxia – target cells are unable to utilise the oxygen, which is being adequately delivered

---

It is most important to recognise that the only category of hypoxia that may be detected by pulse oximetry is hypoxic hypoxia. The other forms of hypoxia will not be indicated by the pulse oximeter if the arterial haemoglobin saturation is satisfactory.

The physiological response to breathing hypoxic atmospheres depends on the duration of the hypoxia. Acute hypoxia of immediate onset has the most devastating effects, which are summarised below. Patients with chronic hypoxia, lasting from hours to many years, and lifelong hypoxia, i.e. those born or living at high altitude, develop compensatory mechanisms allowing them to survive much greater hypoxia than those acutely exposed.

Causes of failure of oxygenation of the blood by the lungs

Low partial pressure of inspired oxygen
High altitude
Hypoxic atmosphere at normal atmospheric pressure

Pulmonary causes
Alveolar hypoventilation:
Chronic bronchitis
Primary alveolar hypoventilation
Airway obstruction
Asthma
Haemothorax or pneumothorax
Drug induced (sedation, neuromuscular blockers)
Sleep apnoea (central and obstructive)

Ventilation–perfusion mismatch:
Chronic bronchitis and emphysema
Multiple emboli
Pneumonia
Atelectasis
Asthma
Pulmonary fibrosis

Reduced surface area for diffusion:
Emphysema
Pulmonary infarction
Pulmonary fibrosis

Alveolar–capillary diffusion defect:
Pulmonary oedema
Adult respiratory distress syndrome
Diffuse pulmonary fibrosis
Lymphangitis carcinomatosa

Cardiovascular causes
Right to left shunt
Cardiac failure

Acute hypoxia

The physiological effects of acute oxygen lack in healthy adults are enumerated in the Box on p. 80.

Neurological features predominate, especially if the oxygen supply diminishes rapidly; consciousness is lost if the supply of oxygen to the brain ceases for more than 10 seconds. The effects of a reduction in oxygen supply to the brain depend on the severity of the reduction. Mild hypoxaemia results in impairment of higher functions, headache, dizziness, restlessness, fatigue, anorexia, impaired night vision and insomnia; moderate hypoxaemia results in behavioural changes, weakness, and decreased sensation to stimuli, including pain; and severe hypoxaemia results in unconsciousness, convulsions and death.[1]

Physiological effects of acute oxygen lack in healthy adults

Cyanosis
Respiratory system:
  Hyperpnoea
  Dyspnoea
  Increased airways resistance

Cardiovascular system:
  Coronary vasodilation
  Systemic vasodilation
  Decreased afterload
  Increased cardiac output
  Increased stroke volume
  Tachycardia
  Systemic hypotension (may rise if hypercapnia coexists)
  Progression to cardiovascular collapse
  Electrocardiogram:
    Inverted T waves
    Slowing of conduction
    Lengthening of P-R interval
    ST elevation
  Capillaries:
    Loss of tone
    Leakage of fluid
  Pulmonary vasoconstriction
  Redistribution of blood flow to coronary, cerebral, and renal arteries

Central nervous system:
  Blood flow to brain increased
  Capillary leakage
  Cerebral oedema
  Raised intracranial pressure
  Damage increased by hypotension and hypercapnia

These effects of hypoxia are only the immediate life-threatening effects. It must be remembered that all cells require sufficient oxygen and will be affected by hypoxia; some cells are more sensitive than others. Cells that are able switch their metabolism to anaerobic pathways, with an increase in lactic acid production and decrease in plasma pH. This occurs whenever cells are supplied with less oxygen than they require and thus incur an oxygen debt. Hypoxia in the unfit patient has a greater detrimental effect and progresses more rapidly than in the fit and well young person.

Referring to complete cessation of oxygenation, Nunn[2] modified Haldane's statement, saying: "Lack of oxygen stops the machine and *then* wrecks the machinery". The organs differ in how long they are able to survive after complete anoxia (cardiac arrest): damage to the cerebral cortex occurs after about one minute, to the heart after five minutes, to the liver and kidney after 10 minutes, and to skeletal muscle after about two hours.

Chronic hypoxia

Acclimatisation to high altitude takes many weeks and is discussed in Chapter 7. Oxygen delivery to the cells is maintained by increasing the haemoglobin concentration, initially by a decrease in plasma volume and then by a much slower increase in red cell mass.[3] These adaptations take place from birth in lifelong high-altitude dwellers.

Respiratory failure

"Respiratory failure" is classified into two subtypes: type 1, the failure to maintain oxygenation; and type 2, hypoxaemia plus hypercapnia.

The pulse oximeter alone will not distinguish between type 1 and type 2. Type 1 respiratory failure is caused by inhalation of hypoxic atmospheres and ventilation–perfusion mismatch. Hyperventilation of an underperfused area of the lungs can eliminate sufficient carbon dioxide, but the blood from the overventilated areas is already fully saturated and therefore cannot compensate for the underventilated areas. Type 1 failure is seen in bronchial asthma, pneumonia, lung fibrosis, pulmonary oedema, pulmonary embolism, septic shock, low cardiac output states, and adult respiratory distress syndrome.

Before the evidence of pulse oximetry is relied on entirely the limitations of the technique must be realised, especially the effect of carboxyhaemoglobin and methaemoglobin. These limitations are dealt with in detail in further chapters.

Normal oxygen saturation as indicated by any oximeter does not necessarily rule out hypoventilation, especially if supplementary oxygen is being given.

As the pulse oximeter is now so widely available there are certain areas in which the use of the technique should be mandatory. Already in many parts of the developed world it is considered negligent not to use a pulse oximeter during anaesthesia. Some other important areas are considered below.

Asthma

Asthma is a common complaint and a common cause of death in children and young adults. Pulse oximetry is an important monitoring technique that should be applied to any patient suffering an acute exacerbation of asthma. Any desaturation that is indicated while the patient is breathing room air should be taken as an indication for admission to hospital. Oxygen should be given in sufficient concentration to raise the SpO_2 and maintain it at $> 95\%$ with humidified oxygen at concentrations of up to 60%. The use of 24% or 28% oxygen is completely inappropriate as these patients will not be compromised by loss of "hypoxic drive". Although the pulse oximeter will give a safe indication of the state of oxygenation of the patient, serial monitoring of arterial blood gases is necessary in a severe attack; if the patient is deteriorating despite conventional bronchodilator treatment, a rise in carbon dioxide is the first indication that mechanical respiratory support is necessary. However, there is often a slight fall in arterial PCO_2 just before a rapid and continuing rise.

Yamamoto et al.[4] have shown that although SpO_2 and peak flow measurements have a limited ability to predict whether hospital admission is necessary, SpO_2 is a valid measure of wheezing severity and is more easily obtained in children of all ages than peak flow measurement.

del Rio Navarro et al.[5] also confirm that pulse oximetry is a useful simple objective method of evaluating asthmatic children, but it is not predictive for a therapeutic decision.

Chronic obstructive pulmonary disease

The terms chronic obstructive pulmonary disease (COPD) and chronic obstructive airway disease (COAD) have become common to indicate a frequent clinical situation formed of a combination of chronic bronchitis, emphysema and airways obstruction. Chronic obstructive pulmonary disease may be a mixture of all three, and the airways obstruction may be fixed or partially reversible. The pulse oximeter is useful in the diagnosis, as a screening instrument and to manage oxygen treatment. However, it is important to remember that if the patient continues to be a smoker the pulse oximeter reading will be a slight overestimation. The amount by which the SpO_2 is higher than the actual oxygen saturation depends on the level of carboxyhaemoglobin circulating; the SpO_2 is approximately equal to (SaO_2 + %HbCO). This is explained in Chapter 11.

There are two discernible patterns of respiratory failure in severe chronic obstructive pulmonary disease, although most patients present with a mixture of symptoms. The patterns differ mainly in the extent to which respiratory drive is preserved as the small airway obstruction progresses. "Pink puffers" (type A) have good respiratory drive and therefore, despite having severe airways obstruction and being very dyspnoeic, maintain good arterial blood gases and normal oxygen saturation. They are usually elderly, cachectic, and exhale through pursed lips (to provide their own positive end-expiratory pressure). "Blue bloaters" (type B) have poor respiratory drive, mild dyspnoea, and less obstruction than type A. They are usually obese and have large volumes of sputum. The arterial blood gases are abnormal, with hypercapnia and hypoxaemia. Because of the hypoxaemia they become polycythaemic. Pulse oximetry on the type B patient shows severe desaturation, often below 85%; saturation is even lower at night, especially during REM (rapid eye movement) sleep.

Before pulse oximetry was available, Trask and Cree[6] showed that all patients with chronic obstructive pulmonary disease who were mildly hypoxic when awake had considerable dips in SaO_2 during sleep. They used a Water's ear oximeter, which was accurate within 5%. The saturation dropped within two to five minutes of falling asleep; it did not drift down slowly. None of their patients had received sedatives, and they were not undergoing acute exacerbations of their disease.

During acute exacerbations of chronic obstructive pulmonary disease, which are usually due to infection, oxygen saturation invariably decreases; the pulse oximeter may be used to indicate improvement or otherwise with antibiotics, bronchodilators and physiotherapy. The pulse oximeter is vitally important in managing oxygen treatment in these patients, although it must be remembered that the partial pressure of arterial carbon dioxide must always be measured in patients sick enough to be hospitalised.

The management of hypoxia in this group of patients is difficult but can be optimised with pulse oximetry. The problem is that those patients with the lowest saturations – the type B, blue bloaters – are already hypercapnic and rely on "hypoxic drive" to keep breathing at all. The addition of uncontrolled amounts of supplementary oxygen may well improve their chronic hypoxaemic state, but at the same time it may worsen their respiratory failure as their hypoxic drive is taken away. It is a truism that patients who really need oxygen often cannot tolerate it, and that those who tolerate oxygen often do not really need it.[7] Thus, hypoxaemia measured by pulse oximetry or arterial blood gas analysis does not necessarily require oxygen treatment. But if the saturation is < 85% and there is profuse sweating, moaning or grunting, then additional oxygen will be required. The $PaCO_2$ should be recorded before treatment. Oxygen should be given to maintain a saturation of at least 85%, and this should be continuously monitored with a pulse oximeter. If the patient was relying on hypoxic drive then the SpO_2 should be allowed to rise just enough to improve the condition clinically, and then maintained at that level. During the acute phase of an exacerbation it may be necessary to infuse a respiratory stimulant such as doxapram intravenously as a form of respiratory drive.

Adult respiratory distress syndrome

Adult respiratory distress syndrome (ARDS) is a severe form of respiratory inadequacy characterised by progressive hypoxaemia; it is refractory to supplemental oxygen. There is tachypnoea and bilateral lung shadowing, which is usually more widespread than straightforward pulmonary oedema. The syndrome is a very serious complication of multiple aetiologies. It still has a mortality of approximately 50%. It is evident from the list of causes (Box) that ideally a pulse oximeter – which is such a cheap and non-invasive technique – should be applied, for continuous monitoring, to any patient suffering from these problems. Any progressive fall in SpO_2 during conventional oxygen treatment should lead to urgent referral to an intensive care unit.

Pulse oximetry for screening

There are several emergency situations in which the pulse oximeter may be used as a screening test to expedite the management of acute problems. The aetiology of acute confusion or delirium is often difficult to determine, but one of the commonest causes of these conditions is hypoxia, which itself may be due to several potentially reversible causes. The application of a pulse oximeter to detect

Causes of adult respiratory distress syndrome

Direct injury to the lungs
Pulmonary contusion
Aspiration of stomach contents
Inhalation of noxious gases or vapours
Near drowning
Pneumonia
Fat embolus
Amniotic fluid embolus
Radiotherapy
Bleomycin

Indirect injury to lungs
Septicaemia
Multiorgan failure
Multiple trauma (extrathoracic)
Hypovolaemic shock
Head injury
Acute pancreatitis
Massive blood transfusion
Diabetic ketoacidosis
Severe burns
Goodpasture's syndrome

hypoxia as a cause is simple, quick, and less distressing to the patient than taking blood for arterial blood gas analysis. Hypoxia sufficient to cause an acute confusional state or worsen an existing one will not necessarily be obvious as cyanosis, especially as this emergency commonly occurs at night. Similarly, hypoxia is a common cause of angina in a patient with pre-existing ischaemic heart disease, and the management of oxygen treatment is greatly simplified by pulse oximetry.

Wagner *et al.*[8] have suggested a simple screening test for respiratory disease in young children. The "88% saturation test" (88%-SAT test) was developed as an alternative to forced peak expiratory flow spirometry in the less cooperative. The subject breathes non-humidified 12% oxygen in nitrogen mixture for 10 minutes, or until the SpO_2 decreases to 88%, whichever occurs first. Abnormal 88%-SAT was defined as a decrease of SpO_2 to 88% within the 10-minute period. They concluded that the 88%-SAT may be more effective than spirometry for identifying reactive airways disease in young uncooperative or developmentally delayed children.

Surgical applications

The viability and condition of extremities and even internal organs may be tested and monitored by pulse oximetry, see Boxon p. 87. A pulse oximeter used for this purpose must show a plethysmogram. Pulse oximetry is *not* a safe method of detecting raised intracompartmental pressure in limbs.[9,10] The probe is placed on the finger or toe of the injured or otherwise compromised limb, and the plethysmogram and oxygen saturation are continuously monitored. Ideally, a second, identical, pulse oximeter should be placed on a non-compromised extremity, although this is not entirely necessary. Both pulse oximeters should indicate the same level of saturation. It is important to know whether the plethysmogram of the pulse oximeter being used for this purpose is "normalised" or not; otherwise, changes in the amplitude, and hence the perfusion, may not be noticed.

Pulse oximetry is a sensitive indicator of perfusion in patients suffering peripheral vascular disease. A comparison of 20 healthy volunteers with 20 patients with peripheral vascular disease showed the technique to be more sensitive than transcutaneous oxygen partial pressure or ankle artery Doppler pressure.[11] Two methods of modified Allen's test, Doppler ultrasound and pulse oximetry, correlated precisely for assessing collateral blood flow to the hand before radial artery cannulation.[12] Pulse oximetry may also be used to assess the cause of a painful hand after an arteriovenous fistula has been created.[13]

Pulse oximetry used for this purpose is only an indication that a pulsatile blood flow exists and what the arterial oxygen saturation is, although it must be remembered that the actual value of SpO_2 in the compromised limb may be normal,[14] and therefore it is only the *plethysmograph* trace that is of use. For measuring the blood flow, Doppler ultrasound is the simplest non-invasive technique, but pulse oximetry provides a method of continuous monitoring.

DeNobile *et al.*[15] validated pulse oximetry as a means of assessing bowel viability at surgery. Segmental intestinal ischaemia was produced in dogs while the saturation indicated by a pulse oximeter on the tongue was compared with the saturation from a second pulse oximeter, the probe of which was on the bowel wall. The segmental ischaemia was increased in steps until there was a sudden fall in saturation or the pulse oximeter on the bowel failed to detect a signal. This was marked on the bowel with a suture and the laparotomy was then closed. On re-exploration at 48 hours, biopsy specimens were taken of normal bowel and at various distances into the ischaemic segment. Necrosis or partial necrosis occurred within 3 cm of the point at which the pulse oximeter warned of poor circulation, but was absent in areas where the pulse oximeter indicated a good circulation.

Monitoring viability with pulse oximetry

Trauma
 Fractures (for example, supracondylar fracture of elbow)
 Vascular injuries to limbs
 Soft tissue injury ("compartment syndromes", crush)

Surgery
 Vascular (atheroma bypass, aortic aneurysm)
 Removal of arterial emboli
 Viability of bowel

Medical
 Dissecting aneurysm

Tollefson *et al.*[16] compared pulse oximetry with Doppler ultrasound and a fluorescent technique for the assessment of bowel viability and found it superior in ease of use, repeatability and interpretation.

A transanal pulse oximeter probe has been used to continuously monitor distal colonic blood flow during aortic reconstruction.[17]

The work on testing the viability of other organs has been purely experimental and has involved the use of reflectance probes. The probe is covered with a suitable sterile flexible plastic bag and may be applied directly to the surface of organs such as the kidney or the brain. This technique is especially useful to assess the blood supply of transplanted organs. During plastic surgery, the pulse oximeter used in this way shows the viability of the blood supply of skin flaps which have been "swung" around, and also of "free" flaps.

Pulse oximetry in the intensive care unit

In most intensive care units and high-dependency units pulse oximetry is used routinely on every patient, whether ventilated[18] or breathing spontaneously. It gives the quickest indication of a fall in arterial oxygen saturation from whatever cause. It is often the first monitoring modality applied on admission to an intensive care unit.

An important use of pulse oximetry in the intensive care unit is the optimisation of oxygen treatment, especially the management of continuous positive airway pressure (CPAP) in the spontaneously

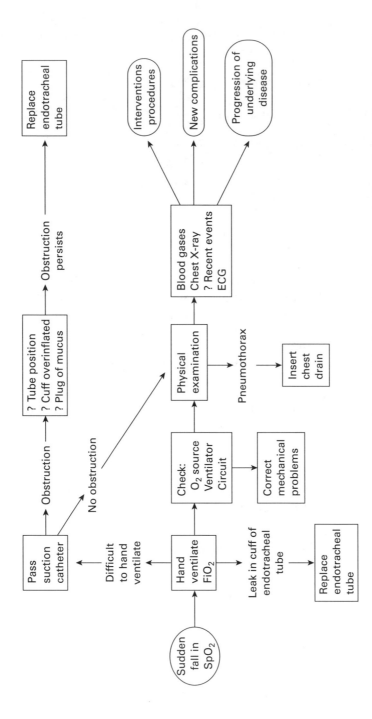

Figure 8.1 Diagnostic algorithm for initial management of acute fall in SpO$_2$ in intensive care unit. Reproduced with permission from the *American Journal of Surgery*.[19]

breathing patient and positive end-expiratory pressure (PEEP) in the mechanically ventilated patient. This must, of course, be done in conjunction with other physiological measurements, such as blood pressure and cardiac output.

It may be useful to have an algorithm, either in writing or in one's mind, about how to manage an acute hypoxic event as detected by pulse oximetry in an intensive care unit. The algorithm in Figure 8.1 is adapted from that of Moore *et al.*[19]

"Routine" pulse oximetry

Should the pulse oximeter be as essential in the routine examination as a patella hammer, an ophthalmoscope or a non-invasive blood pressure monitor? Two issues, appropriate scientific application and medical economics, bear on this.[20] Even experienced physicians are inaccurate in their estimation of arterial oxygenation, and moderate to severe anaemia makes the estimation impossible.[21] Already, electronic devices are replacing the clinical thermometer and the manual sphygmomanometer, more for convenience than for efficiency or accuracy. The pulse oximeter offers an objective estimation of arterial oxygenation that is cheap, reliable and non-invasive. As Neff[20] pointed out, a fall of 5% from 96% to 91% is unlikely to be noticeable clinically but is often very important. The pulse oximeter is also important for optimising oxygen treatment. Neff advocates its routine use in pulmonary disease; I believe that its use should be more widespread, and that pulse oximetry should form part of any clinical investigation where there is the remotest risk of hypoxaemia.

References

1 Cade JF, Pain MCF. *Essentials of respiratory medicine*. Oxford: Blackwell Scientific, 1988.
2 Nunn JF. *Applied respiratory physiology*. 3rd edn. London: Butterworths, 1987.
3 Ward MP, Milledge JS, West JB. *High altitude medicine and physiology*. London: Chapman & Hall, 1989.
4 Yamamoto LG, Wiebe RA, Anaya C *et al*. Pulse oximetry and peak flow as indicators of wheezing severity in children and improvement following bronchodilator treatments. *Am J Emerg Med* 1992;**10**:519–24.
5 del Rio Navarro BE, Briseno Perez C, Sienra Monge JJ, Prieto Urza L, Predes Novelo C, Carrillo H. Clinical usefulness of pulse oximetry in asthmatic children. *Rev Alg Mex* 1994;**41**:110–14.

6 Trask CH, Cree EM. Oximeter studies on patients with chronic obstructive emphysema, awake and asleep. *N Engl J Med* 1962;**266**: 639–42.

7 Brewis RAL. *Lecture notes on respiratory medicine.* Oxford: Blackwell Scientific, 1991.

8 Wagner CL, Brooks JG, Richter SE, Pratt K, Phelps DL. The "88% saturation test": a simple lung function test for young children. *Pediatrics* 1994;**93**:63–7.

9 Mars M, Hadley GP. Failure of pulse oximetry in the assessment of raised limb intracompartmental pressure. *Injury* 1994;**25**:379–81.

10 Mars M, Maseko S, Thomson SR, Rout C. Can pulse oximetry detect raised intracompartmental pressure? *S Afr J Surg* 1994;**32**:48–50.

11 Joyce WP, Walsh K, Gough JB *et al.* Pulse oximetry: a new non-invasive assessment of peripheral arterial occlusive disease. *Br J Surg* 1990; **77**:115–7.

12 Pillow K, Herrick IA. Pulse oximetry compared with Doppler ultrasound for assessment of collateral blood flow to the hand. *Anaesthesia* 1991; **46**:388–90.

13 Halevy A, Halpern Z, Negri M *et al.* Pulse oximetry in the evaluation of the painful hand after arteriovenous fistula creation. *J Vasc Surg* 1991; **14**:537–9.

14 Liisberg-Larsen OC, Schroeder TV. Pulse oximetry for the assessment of lower extremity ischaemia. *Ugeskr Laeger* 1993;**155**:2139–41.

15 DeNobile J, Guzzetta P, Patterson K. Pulse oximetry as a means of assessing bowel viability. *J Surg Res* 1990;**48**:21–3.

16 Tollefson DF, Wright DJ, Reddy DJ, Kitanar EB. Intraoperative determination of intestinal viability by pulse oximetry. *Ann Vasc Surg* 1995;**9**:357–60.

17 Gardner GP, LaMorte WW, Obi-Tabot ET, Menzoian JO. Transanal intracolonic pulse oximetry as a means of monitoring the adequacy of colonic perfusion. *J Surg Res* 1994;**57**:537–40.

18 Jubran A, Tobin MJ. Reliability of pulse-oximetry in titrating supplemental oxygen therapy in ventilator dependent patients. *Chest* 1990;**97**:1420–5.

19 Moore FA, Haenel JB, Moore EE, Abernathy CM. Hypoxic events in the surgical intensive care unit. *Am J Surg* 1990;**160**:647–51.

20 Neff TA. Routine oximetry – a fifth vital sign? *Chest* 1988;**94**:227.

21 Comroe JH, Botelho S. The unreliability of cyanosis in the recognition of arterial anoxemia. *Am J Med Sci* 1947;**214**:1–6.

9: Specific clinical applications

9.1 Emergency medicine

Anaesthetists were quick to see the enormous benefit to the safety of the patient of using pulse oximeters, and doctors, nurses and medical technicians involved in emergency care soon recognised the advantages of pulse oximetry over purely clinical assessment of oxygenation. Pulse oximeters are now regularly used in accident and emergency departments, and also in the prehospital care of the sick and injured.

In this area, however, it cannot be emphasised enough that pulse oximetry can be safely used only if the limitations of the technique are realised by all users (see Chapter 10). Failure to recognise hypoxaemia has been identified as one of the major avoidable causes of death in trauma patients.[1] Studies show that hypoxaemia regularly goes unrecognised,[2] especially in patients who are not complaining of respiratory distress.[3] Key points that must be remembered by all users, but especially those working in emergency medicine, are shown in the Box.

Key points in use of pulse oximeters
- Pulse oximeters are calibrated for adult haemoglobin (HbA)
- Pulse oximeters must not be used with patients suspected of having inhaled carbon monoxide (this includes attempted suicide, and those involved in conflagrations or in road accidents involving fire or inhalation of exhaust fumes)
- Pulse oximeters must not be used with patients suspected of having other abnormal haemoglobins (for example methaemoglobin)
- Pulse oximeters do not indicate the adequacy of ventilation, especially if supplementary oxygen is being given
- There is a non-linear relationship between SpO_2 and oxygen partial pressure (PaO_2) which depends on the oxyhaemoglobin dissociation curve (see Chapter 6). The curve may also be "shifted" by the disease state of the patient – for example, to the left by blood transfusion or to the right by sickle cell anaemia

---

The effect of circulating carboxyhaemoglobin is discussed in Chapter 11. Haemoglobin has a very high affinity for carbon monoxide, and the problem with the conventional pulse oximeter is that even minimal amounts of carboxyhaemoglobin make the pulse oximeter overestimate the oxygen saturation. The indicated SpO_2 is approximately equal to the percentage oxygen saturation plus the percentage of carboxyhaemoglobin. Even small doses of carbon monoxide therefore often make the pulse oximeter read 100%. It must be considered negligent for a pulse oximeter to be attached to any patient who has been involved in even the smallest of conflagrations or has suffered burns. Heavy smokers and those whose work consists of driving in inner cities will also have raised concentrations of carboxyhaemoglobin (see Chapter 11).

Methaemoglobinaemia causes less danger in that, as the concentration of methaemoglobin increases, so the indicated saturation tends to 85%. When the oxygen saturation is greater than 85%, no harm is likely to come to the patient by this inaccuracy. However, if the patient is also hypoxaemic, with an oxygen saturation < 85%, a false sense of their wellbeing will be given by the pulse oximeter.

Prehospital care: road traffic accidents

Those involved in emergency care need to remember that adequate oxygenation does not necessarily equate with adequate ventilation and adequate elimination of carbon dioxide. This is especially the case when supplementary oxygen is given. In 1989, a general practitioner advocated the indiscriminate use of pulse oximetry at roadside accidents. He suggested erroneously that measuring oxygen saturation with a pulse oximeter may indicate the first signs of hypoventilation, but most of his patients were receiving supplementary oxygen or 50% oxygen plus 50% nitrous oxide (Entonox).[4] Further, many trapped patients have received small amounts of carbon monoxide, and even such small amounts will produce significant concentrations of carboxyhaemoglobin.[5] It has also been suggested that pulse oximetry gives an indication of tissue oxygenation.[6] Fully saturated oxyhaemoglobin with a low cardiac output may produce a high value of SpO_2, but with tissue hypoxia.[7]

Prehospital care: medical emergencies

Several studies of the usefulness of pulse oximetry in the prehospital care of medical emergencies have been carried out in the United States. Of 62 consecutive critically ill patients, 15 had saturations below 91%, and pulse oximetry detected two patients with saturations below 80% who were otherwise undetected. In both of these cases prehospital intervention by paramedics, based on the evidence provided by the pulse oximeter, improved the patient's condition. These authors warn of erroneous readings due to abnormal haemoglobins and motion artefacts, and also possible failure due to severe hypotension, anaemia, peripheral vasoconstriction, or optical interference.[8] Another study with similar results suggests that pulse oximetry is a very useful monitor of oxygenation so long as the physiology (Chapter 6) and limitations (Chapter 10) are fully understood.[9]

The importance of prehospital pulse oximetry is confirmed by a recent study in which 14 of 50 patients were found to be hypoxic (oxygen saturation < 90% for longer than one minute) *en route* to hospital; only four had been clinically recognised as hypoxic.[10]

Pulse oximetry in the accident and emergency department

The role of pulse oximetry in the accident and emergency department is varied and includes routine monitoring of acutely ill patients; monitoring oxygenation of patients undergoing minor procedures under some form of sedation; and discrete oxygen saturation measurements instead of arterial blood gas sample analysis.

When a pulse oximeter was applied to a series of patients presenting as medical emergencies to a large city hospital, 42% were found to be unexpectedly hypoxaemic – that is, with oxygen saturations of 94% or less. With a normal oxyhaemoglobin dissociation curve, this represents an arterial partial pressure of oxygen of less than 10 kPa.

Maneker *et al.*[11] have shown that children with respiratory illness presenting to an accident department should be assessed with pulse oximetry, as clinical observation usually underestimated the severity of hypoxaemia. This has been reinforced by Mower *et al.*,[12] who consider pulse oximetry to be a "fifth pediatric vital sign".

All patients who have been sedated should be monitored with, at least, pulse oximetry. This has become evident from studies on patients undergoing fibreoptic gastrointestinal endoscopy (see later) and has recently been confirmed by Wright,[13] who looked at 27 patients in an accident and emergency department requiring sedation with benzodiazepines with or without opioids. They were monitored with capnography and pulse oximetry. The capnometer was attached to the patient with a nasal probe to monitor the end-tidal carbon dioxide (this is approximately equivalent to the arterial carbon dioxide partial pressure). Pulse oximetry was with a finger probe. Observations were continued for two hours after the procedure. The average end-tidal carbon dioxide increased from 35·9 mmHg to 42·1 mmHg and the oxygen saturation on average fell from a baseline of 98% to 94%, but eight patients became significantly hypoxic and hypercapnic. In none of these patients was the hypoxaemia noticed clinically without the pulse oximeter.[13]

Pulse oximetry should also be used during procedures without sedation in which the airway is "shared" or may be compromised. Tracheal suction and gastric lavage both cause transient hypoxaemia.[14]

Applying a pulse oximeter to the fingers or toes of an injured limb is a good indicator of the oxygenation of the limb and of proximal arterial injury.[14] Continuous monitoring with a pulse oximeter may also provide early indication of a compartment syndrome complicating a closed limb fracture.[15]

One major advantage of pulse oximetry is that, for patients who require only measurement of their arterial oxygen, the technique is non-invasive, quick and painless. In a study in Memphis involving 20 000 patients over a period of four months, 699 arterial blood samples were taken for formal blood gas and acid–base analysis during the first two months. During the second two-month period pulse oximetry was available; arterial blood sampling was reduced to 440 patients with the same explicit criteria. This 37% decrease was due to fewer samples being taken when only an assessment of oxygenation was required.[16] Pulse oximetry in the accident and emergency department saves time and money and allows arterial oxygenation to be assessed in the majority rather than the minority of patients.

9.2 Anaesthesia

Although originally developed for the respiratory physiologist, the pulse oximeter is most often and most importantly used when anaesthesia is given. It could even be said that the pulse oximeter is the ultimate safety monitor in the operating theatre and anaesthetic room, as it ensures that the anaesthetist is aware of any decrease in oxygenation; it is "failsafe" in that there must be a pulsatile blood flow for its operation. Thus it warns of failure of either oxygenation or circulation. The pulse oximeter is now considered, in most countries, to be one of the basic items of monitoring equipment that should be used during every anaesthetic.

The level of cyanosis detectable by experienced clinicians varies between individuals and with changes in ambient lighting.[17] As pulse oximeters become more and more common they should be used whenever possible, from the moment patients enter the operating facility until they are fully conscious.

Causes of perioperative hypoxaemia

A reduction in arterial oxygen saturation from the ideal during anaesthesia, surgery or recovery has numerous causes. Arterial desaturation may be due to diminished alveolar oxygen tension or an increase in the difference in oxygen tension between the alveolus and the blood in the pulmonary artery ($P_{(A-a)}O_2$). The causes of a reduction

---

Causes of reduced alveolar partial pressure (P_AO_2) associated with anaesthesia

Diminished inspired oxygen pressure (P_iO_2)
  Flow meter error
  Zero oxygen flow
  Volatile agent vaporised in air
  Diffusion hypoxia

Diminished alveolar ventilation
  Central respiratory depression
    Neurological disease
    Premedication
    Anaesthetic agent
  Peripheral respiratory depression
    Neuromuscular disease
    Neuromuscular blocking drugs
  Increased respiratory deadspace
    Drugs
    Intermittent positive-pressure ventilation (IPPV)
    Hypotension
    Cardiopulmonary disease
    Anaesthesia breathing system
  Mechanical impairment
  Airway obstruction
    Oropharyngeal soft tissue
    Regurgitated stomach contents
    Uncleared secretions
    Foreign body
    Respiratory disease
  Thoracic wall
    Bone and joint disease
    Posture or immobilisation
    Surgical retraction, packing etc.

in alveolar partial pressure and those of an increased difference are shown in the Box.[18] Most of these causes are self-explanatory.

Lack of an adequate flow of oxygen in the required concentration to the anaesthetic machine is an obvious and common cause of hypoxaemia under anaesthesia. The causes are numerous and include blocks in the flow meter, misreading of the flow meter, and leaks in the anaesthetic machine and the breathing system. The inspired oxygen concentration should be monitored at all times.

The use of air as the carrier gas has all but disappeared from modern anaesthesia, but it is still used in the developing world where high-quality cylinder oxygen is expensive or unobtainable. Volatile anaesthetic agents can be given safely with air as the carrier gas by using drawover apparatus such as the EMO vaporiser or Penlon TriService apparatus (Penlon, Abingdon, Oxfordshire), but whenever possible supplemental oxygen should be given by using the attachments provided with this equipment. When cylinder oxygen is not available, an oxygen concentrator should be used.

Diffusion hypoxia

Nitrous oxide is approximately 40 times more soluble in blood than nitrogen. Theoretically, when an atmosphere of oxygen and nitrous oxide is suddenly replaced by an atmosphere of oxygen and nitrogen, the nitrous oxide diffusing out of the blood passes through the lungs faster than the nitrogen diffusing in the opposite direction. If the inspired oxygen from the oxygen–nitrogen mixture is only 21%, then the concentration of oxygen may be diluted below a safe level. This is known as diffusion hypoxia. Because of this theoretical possibility it is always prudent to give > 40% oxygen for 10 minutes after nitrous oxide is stopped.

The validity of this recommendation has been investigated recently by Brodsky et al.[19] Sixty healthy patients, ASA class I or II, were divided into two groups. Fifty patients received an anaesthetic containing nitrous oxide and oxygen in a 3:2 ratio, with isoflurane, and 10 patients received oxygen and isoflurane only. All patients were breathing spontaneously. At the end of the operation the gases were abruptly replaced by room air. The arterial oxygen saturation was continuously monitored with a pulse oximeter. The patients given nitrous oxide and oxygen showed a fall in SpO_2 of approximately 4% within three minutes of stopping the mixture.

The patients whose anaesthetic was composed of oxygen and isoflurane showed no significant fall below preoperative values until 4·5 minutes after changing to room air. The two groups did not differ after five minutes. Three patients in the nitrous oxide and oxygen group had significant hypoxic episodes (< 30 seconds of < 90% SpO_2); in each case this was due to respiratory obstruction, which was quickly corrected by changing the position of the patient's head.[19] Although this degree of desaturation is tolerated well by healthy patients, it must still be recommended that to avoid risk of hypoxaemia 100% oxygen be given immediately on stopping any anaesthetic. This is especially important in patients with cardiovascular or respiratory disease, but also in healthy patients, as they may experience airway obstruction, coughing or breath-holding when awaking from general anaesthesia.

Diminished alveolar ventilation

Diminished alveolar ventilation, which causes both hypercapnia and hypoxaemia, may be caused by respiratory depression, increased respiratory dead space, or mechanical impairment to respiration.

Central neurological disease leading to respiratory depression is uncommon except for raised intracranial pressure and the effects of certain drugs. The respiratory control centres are in the pons and the medulla. Any increase in the pressure of cerebrospinal fluid or direct pressure on these areas results in their depression; as the cranium is rigid, space-occupying lesions or oedema in any part of the brain may lead to respiratory depression. Uncommon causes of hypoventilation are Ondine's curse (see later) and the Pickwickian syndrome. The pickwickian syndrome (primary alveolar hypoventilation) is characterised by a combination of obesity, episodic somnolence, hypoventilation, hypercapnia, cyanosis, polycythaemia and pulmonary hypertension with right ventricular failure. It is thought to have a central neurological origin.

Most analgesics and anaesthetics cause a degree of central respiratory depression. The depressant effects of the opioids are well known, and respiratory depression is common after quite modest doses of benzodiazepines or any other sedative, including alcohol. Intravenous anaesthetics given as a bolus often cause a brief apnoeic period, and subsequent doses or infusions cause central respiratory depression.

The volatile anaesthetics depress the respiratory centre (although diethyl ether has a stimulant effect at low to moderate clinical concentrations). These depressant effects cause a rise in arterial carbon dioxide owing to hypoventilation, but the hypoxic effect may not be apparent if increased concentrations of oxygen are given. The presence of another anaesthetic gas or vapour may actually improve oxygenation during the first few minutes of administration by the second gas effect. For example, during the first few breaths of a mixture of nitrous oxide and oxygen, the uptake of nitrous oxide initially exceeds that of oxygen, therefore the alveolar concentration of oxygen is higher than that being supplied to the patient.

Neuromuscular disease will always cause hypoventilation in the spontaneously breathing anaesthetised patient. Many patients with such mainly hereditary problems live on the verge of respiratory failure and decompensate with anaesthesia, as may those with myasthenia gravis. Patients with thoracic malignancy, either primary or metastatic, may have the Eaton–Lambert myasthenic syndrome. Hypokalaemia and hypophosphataemia also weaken normally healthy voluntary muscle.

Neuromuscular blocking drugs obviously lead to gross respiratory depression. It must be borne in mind that other drugs may interfere with neuromuscular conduction – for example polymyxin, neomycin, streptomycin and kanamycin.

Despite many investigations, the actual cause of increase in the difference between the partial pressure of oxygen between the alveolar gas and arterial blood ($P_{(A-a)}O_2$) has not been found,[20] although several suggestions have been made (Box).[18]

Possible causes of increased $P_{(A-a)}O_2$

- Impaired diffusion
- Increased intrapulmonary shunt (venous admixture)
- Increased scatter of ventilation–perfusion ratios
- Increased inspired oxygen concentration
- Decreased mixed venous oxygen tension
- Shift of oxyhaemoglobin dissociation curve

Diffusion of oxygen may be impaired by pulmonary congestion or oedema, which increases the length of the diffusion pathway for oxygen in the pulmonary capillaries. The capillary transit time will be reduced by increased cardiac output, as in anaemia or other causes of a hyperdynamic circulation, giving less time for the blood in the capillaries to equilibrate with alveolar gas. The total area of alveolar–capillary membrane may be reduced by disease, but perioperatively the most likely cause is surgical removal of all or part of a lung.

Intrapulmonary shunt or venous admixture refers to the bypass of some of the desaturated mixed venous blood direct to the end capillary blood in the lungs. The shunt, which is normally < 2% of the cardiac output, constitutes the venous drainage from the bronchi and the thebesian veins. To this anatomical shunt may be added a pathological shunt which embraces mixed venous blood that has passed through unventilated areas of the lungs – for example atelectasis and bronchial obstruction. Further shunting may be caused by right to left shunting in congenital heart disease.

Under ideal conditions, exactly the right amount of blood should perfuse each area of the lungs for the ventilation in that area. Even in healthy young adults this ventilation–perfusion ratio is not perfect, mainly because of the effect of gravity. During surgery, under either general anaesthesia or regional block with sedation, the ventilation–perfusion ratio deteriorates owing to a combination of anatomical positioning, anaesthesia itself, and surgical retraction.

Reduction of hypoxaemia by pulse oximetry

Hypoxaemia has been shown to be much more common in the anaesthetic room, operating theatre and recovery areas than originally assumed.[5,7,8] Moller et al.[21] in Denmark observed 296 patients chosen at random; patients with a history of severe lung disease and a preoperative oxygen saturation < 90% were excluded. The anaesthetics were given by experienced anaesthetists. Two anaesthetists were present at each procedure, one giving the anaesthetic but unable to observe the pulse oximeter, and the other observing the pulse oximeter. One or more episodes of mild hypoxaemia (SpO_2 86–90%) occurred in 53% of patients; episodes of severe hypoxaemia (SpO_2 < 81%) were recorded in 20% of patients. The mild hypoxaemic episodes lasted up to 34·6 minutes (mean 2·3 minutes) and 70% of these episodes were not detected by the anaesthetist giving the anaesthetic. In the remaining 30% the anaesthetist diagnosed hypoxaemia with a mean delay of 70 seconds, and after a mean period of 57 seconds the SpO_2 was indicated as being > 90%. The authors concluded that hypoxaemic episodes are common, and that preoxygenation and supplemental oxygen are required in all patients until full arousal postoperatively.[21]

In a further study Moller et al. investigated how great a difference pulse oximetry makes to the frequency and depth of hypoxaemic episodes related to general anaesthesia. Two hundred adult patients were randomised into two groups. In one group, pulse oximeter data and alarms were available to the anaesthesia team, but in the other the SpO_2 and alarms were available only to an observer. The incidence of hypoxaemia was much reduced in the first group. The second group had 47 recorded episodes with SpO_2 of 86–90%, 10 of 81–85%, 5 of 76–80%, and 5 of < 76%. The first group had 22 episodes of 86–90% and 5 of 76–80%, with no recordings < 75%. The differences between the two groups were even greater in the recovery room.[22]

Hypoxaemia at induction

Several studies have shown how easily patients become desaturated around the time of induction of anaesthesia. This is the most critical time of a general anaesthetic because of the side effects of the induction agents, the onset of neuromuscular blockade, loss of protective reflexes, mechanical problems with the airway, respiratory depression, and difficulty with tracheal intubation. Although the level of arousal of the anaesthetist is at its highest at this time, concentration on just one of these occurrences may take all his or her attention and it is therefore important that the pulse oximeter is applied before any drugs are given.

Ideally, all patients should be preoxygenated before induction of anaesthesia. Unless high concentrations of oxygen are given by manual positive-pressure ventilation immediately after consciousness is lost, significant hypoxaemia will occur within one minute, even in the fittest patient, and particularly with obese patients. The mean oxygen saturation in patients studied by Drummond and Park fell from 96% before induction to 85% one minute after induction and administration of suxamethonium, unless the patients had been preoxygenated. Surprisingly, haemoglobin concentration, forced expiratory volume in one second, forced vital capacity, age and smoking habit were not related to the degree of arterial desaturation. The hypoxaemia was worse than expected (mean of 80%) at one minute when the patient was obese.[23] This work was carried out using a Hewlett-Packard ear oximeter, the accuracy of which is disturbed by carboxyhaemoglobin; the effects of smoking on the desaturation may have been erroneous in this study as carboxyhaemoglobin makes spectrophotometric techniques calibrated for adult haemoglobin overread. This would also occur with pulse oximetry (see Chapter 11).

Benumof et al.[24] compared the time taken for recovery from 1 mg/kg of suxamethonium to theoretical time to desaturation with initial $F_AO_2 = 0.87$. The results are shown in Figure 9.1.

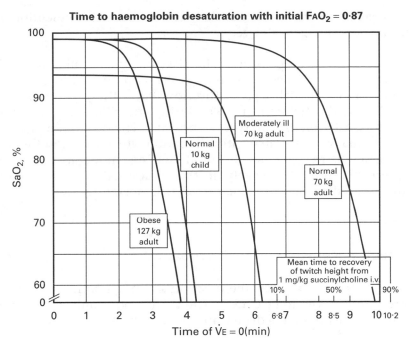

Figure 9.1 SaO$_2$ versus time of apnoea for various types of patient.

To elucidate preoxygenation further, Drummond and Park assessed four different groups. Patients in group I were preoxygenated for one minute by breathing normally through a tightly fitting mask and a Mapleson A breathing system supplied with oxygen at 10 l/min. Those in group II received the same preoxygenation but with a standardised simulated leak (9·5 mm diameter hole in the mask opposite the mouth).

Patients in group III were supplied with oxygen as group I, but were instructed to inhale maximally and then exhale maximally three times, after which anaesthesia was induced. Group IV subjects were not preoxygenated, but the lungs were inflated manually three times with oxygen by compression of the reservoir bag immediately after induction of anaesthesia. Oxygen saturation was recorded before induction and at one, two and three minutes after induction. The mean saturation after three minutes was 96·8% in group I, 93·6% in group II, and 98% in group III. In group IV, measurements were stopped at two minutes, when the mean saturations had fallen to 92·9%. This study concluded that three vital capacity breaths of oxygen from the reservoir bag are adequate and acceptable for

101

preoxygenation in healthy, ASA I and II patients presenting for routine non-emergency surgery.[23]

In Kong et al's[25] comparison of the risks of hypoxaemia during the induction phase in neonates and small infants in a district general hospital and a specialist paediatric hospital, a third of the patients experienced desaturation of > 5% during induction. There was no difference between the two types of hospital. The highest incidence of hypoxaemia was associated with intubation while awake. In the non-specialist district general hospital setting moderate to severe hypoxaemia was more likely if the anaesthetist present during induction did not have a regular paediatric operating list.[25]

Correct placement of endotracheal tube

It is, of course, vital that the position of the endotracheal tube is correct and proved to be correct. The correct positioning of the tube should be checked immediately after insertion (Box).

Checking the position of the endotracheal tube

- Observation of chest wall movement with positive airway pressure
- Auscultation
- Capnography
- Pulse oximetry

Capnometry has been said to be the best method to confirm the placement of a tracheal tube,[26] and pulse oximetry may provide only a very late indication of oesophageal intubation. The delay is caused mainly by preoxygenation, as this may prevent hypoxaemia for several minutes in the event of no respiratory movement in the lungs.[27] Recent work confirms that capnography is a more rapid indicator of oesophageal intubation.[28] When capnography is used, oesophageal intubation may be detected with the first respiratory cycle. The pulse oximeter does not show a decrease in SpO_2 for at least 30 seconds if the patient has a fractional inspired oxygen (F_iO_2) of 1·0 during preoxygenation. This delay is shortened to < 10 seconds if the F_iO_2 was 0·3 or less during preventilation. Pulse oximetry is no substitute for capnography in detecting inadvertent oesophageal intubation. If there is no capnograph, however, or if the capnograph undergoes technical failure, the position of the tracheal tube may be confirmed by observing the SpO_2 for a prolonged period while giving 100% oxygen; there should be no reduction in oxygen saturation.[29]

A tracheal tube correctly inserted through the larynx may be advanced too far, entering a main bronchus or even the right lower lobe bronchus. This should be easily detected by observation and auscultation and cannot be detected with a pulse oximeter. Barker et al.[30] compared the ability to detect endobronchial intubation of three types of oxygen monitor: pulse oximeter, transcutaneous oxygen tension monitor, and an experimental fibreoptic intra-arterial monitor of oxygen tension. The pulse oximeter showed negligible change in oxygen saturation during endobronchial intubation, with inspired oxygen fractions > 0·3. Simultaneous oxygen tensions decreased by 42–64% with the transcutaneous device, and by 64–79% with the fibreoptic system. The decrease in oxygen tension was maximal at two minutes, the experimental fibreoptic system being marginally faster.[30]

The laryngeal mask

The introduction of the laryngeal mask has made a considerable change to anaesthetic practice – in many centres it is used for virtually all anaesthetics where previously a mask, with or without a Guedel airway, would have been routine. This change has meant that there is an increased risk of desaturation at the time of induction of anaesthesia.

Haynes et al.[31] randomised 87 healthy adult patients: 12 received no preoxygenation; 25 received partial denitrogenation by breathing oxygen from the start of the injection of the induction agent; and 25 received formal denitrogenation by breathing oxygen for three minutes before induction. A further 25 patients received five "tidal volume" breaths immediately after induction of anaesthesia. Pulse oximetry showed significant desaturation (mean SpO_2 = 89·5%) at 60 seconds in the group that was not given any supplementary oxygen. There was no significant desaturation in either of the two groups that were preoxygenated (mean SpO_2 = 98% at one minute), and there was a fall to a mean of 93% in the group that had the five tidal volume breaths of oxygen after induction. This study concluded that partial or full denitrogenation should be performed in all patients in whom anaesthesia is to be induced with fentanyl and propofol with subsequent laryngeal mask insertion, and that manual ventilation at induction of anaesthesia was not effective in preventing hypoxaemia.[31]

Delay in detection of impending disaster

It is easy to become reliant upon the pulse oximeter as the ultimate safety monitor in anaesthesia, but it must always be remembered that there will be a delay following some mechanical misadventure before the alarm on the pulse oximeter sounds. The response time of the less sensitive instruments may be doubled or trebled if the blood flow is reduced by venous congestion or hypothermia, either peripheral or central.[32]

Verhoeff and Sykes[33] simulated a number of situations during anaesthesia that would lead to arterial hypoxaemia, using the MacPuf computer model of the cardiorespiratory system. The situations, which were based on a 70 kg paralysed patient, were: disconnection from the breathing system; oxygen supply failure with continued mechanical ventilation; disconnection of fresh gas supply to Mapleson D system; and disconnection of fresh gas supply to circle absorption system. The simulations were for an oxygen consumption of 250 ml/min and a carbon dioxide production of 200 ml/min, ventilated with a tidal volume of 500 ml at 12 breaths/min. The fresh gas oxygen concentration was 30%. The simulations showed appreciable differences between the rate of arterial desaturation resulting from each of the four types of oxygen supply failure. For example, in the case of loss of fresh gas supply to circle absorption system with a patient whose functional residual capacity was 3l, the SpO_2 would not fall below 90% for six minutes, compared with less than one minute for complete disconnection of the patient from the breathing system.[33]

Gruber et al.[34] found that 95% of patients placed on oxygen attained equilibration of SpO_2 within 3·5 minutes. Most (95%) patients taken off supplemental oxygen attained equilibration within 4·5 minutes.

Cook et al.[35] investigated the length of delay of several monitoring modes before the alarm sounded to either a disconnect event or a loss of oxygen event. Using monitors with alarms for the variables, shown in Table 9.2.1, they measured the times before each led to an alarm. The work was done on 30 kg pigs which were anaesthetised, paralysed and ventilated.

Regional analgesia

It is easy to become unaware of hypoxaemia when the patient is having surgery under some form of regional analgesia. For several

Table 9.2.1 Length of delay before the alarm[35]

Seconds after event	Loss of O_2 event		Disconnect event	
	Variable	Change	Variable	Change
< 30			F_iO_2	40 → 20%
			$ETCO_2$	41 → 0 mmHg
30	F_iO_2	36 → 26%	PaO_2	164 → 138 mmHg
	PaO_2	138 → 113 mmHg	SpO_2	97 → 82%
			TcO_2	83 → 58 mmHg
60	TcO_2	68 → 47 mmHg	$PaCO_2$	49 → 72 mmHg
90	SpO_2	98 → 70%	$TcCO_2$	89 → 112 mmHg
			EEG	10 → 5 Hz
120			Arterial pressure	98 → 83 mmHg
225			Heart rate	122 → 90 beats/min
240	EEG	9 → 5 Hz		
	Arterial pressure	116 → 96 mmHg		
	Heart rate	94 → 119 beats/min		
300	Pulmonary artery pressure	17 → 30 mmHg	Pulmonary artery pressure	15 → 30 mm Hg
360	$TcCO_2$	68 → 47 mmHg		
390	$ETCO_2$	41 → 34 mmHg		
420	$PaCO_2$	46 → 35 mmHg		

reasons it is important to monitor oxygen saturation during such procedures.

It is common to use regional anaesthesia to sedate patients undergoing surgical procedures. Many of these patients have surgery under a conduction block because they are considered to be at risk with general anaesthesia; this is often because of poor respiratory function or reserve. To make the procedure more pleasant for the patient, intravenous sedation with, for example, midazolam, diazepam or propofol is given. Some anaesthetists routinely give supplementary oxygen during such procedures, and this seems prudent. A trial to ascertain whether supplementary oxygen was necessary had to be abandoned when three-quarters of the patients to whom no added oxygen was given had significant desaturation (SpO_2 75–88%) when mildly sedated with midazolam.[36] The risk of upper airway obstruction is much higher in the sedated patient, however mild the sedation. It must be remembered that snoring is upper airway obstruction.

> **Causes of hypoxaemia during regional analgesia**
> - Concomitant sedation
> - Positioning of the patient and drapes
> - Effects of the regional blockade itself

Desaturation may, in the unfit patient, be due to the way the patient has been positioned on the operating table. This may be due to discomfort in unanaesthetised areas of the body, obesity, congestive cardiac failure, or other causes of orthopnoea. Drapes covering the face are also potent causes of hypoxia.

The regional conduction block itself may leave the compromised patient with a mechanical disadvantage to respiration. The most obvious scenario is the intradural or extradural blockade, which intentionally or otherwise blocks intercostal musculature in the patient, who relies on intercostal movements to a greater extent than the fit adult at rest. The ultimate extension of this is the "total spine", when the roots of the phrenic nerves are included in the block.

During lumbar epidural or spinal anaesthesia the pulse oximeter may be more reliable if the probe is placed on a toe, as the pulse amplitude may be greater due to vasodilatation.[37] This, of course, will not be the case with peripheral vascular disease.

9.3 Postoperative recovery

The period between the end of surgery and when the patient is fully conscious is when hypoxaemia is most likely to go unnoticed. Until recently, this was the time when the most junior member of the operating theatre staff was left, unsupported, to look after the patient. The dangers to a patient's wellbeing are now recognised to the extent that special postgraduate qualifications have become available for nursing staff specialising in this work. By far the greatest risk during this period is respiratory failure, varying from mild and unnoticeable insufficiency to respiratory arrest. Many patients have some degree of peripheral circulatory shutdown, so that mild degrees of desaturation go unnoticed. For these reasons, the pulse oximeter must be regarded as the most important item of monitoring technology during the postoperative recovery phase.

During the early 1950s arterial desaturation during and after open chest surgery, with postoperative hypoxaemia, was reported, and this was sometimes regarded as peculiar to that specialty. In the early 1960s, however, postoperative hypoxaemia was found to occur after even the most trivial surgical procedures performed under general anaesthesia.[38]

Some of the criteria that apply to anaesthesia also apply to the postoperative period, and some of what is said here is a repetition but with a bias towards the staff involved in the postoperative recovery area.

Two recent developments have highlighted the problem of postoperative hypoxaemia. First, 20 years ago operating theatres were usually single, with an associated anaesthetic room and small recovery area close by. Modern theatre suites or complexes have 4–12 adjacent theatres, each with its own anaesthetic room but with one large recovery facility. Thus there may be some delay between the patient being disconnected from high concentrations of oxygen on the operating table and subsequent arrival in the recovery room and readministration of supplementary oxygen. The second development has been the introduction of portable pulse oximeters, which have provided a convenient non-invasive portable method of monitoring oxygen saturation continuously from induction to full recovery.[39]

It is important to remember that pulse oximetry indicates the level of oxygen in the blood; it does not warn of mild degrees of respiratory insufficiency, especially if supplementary oxygen is being given. Mild degrees of respiratory failure lead to increased carbon dioxide concentration in the alveolar gas displacing oxygen and therefore decreasing the concentration of oxygen, furthering hypoxia. Thus, mild degrees of respiratory failure will be indicated by a fall in SpO_2, provided the patient is breathing air.

A simplified list of the causes of hypoxaemia specific to the recovery period is shown in the Box and elucidated below.

Causes of postoperative hypoxaemia
- Upper airway obstruction
- Bronchospasm
- Reduction in functional residual capacity
- Ventilation–perfusion imbalance
- Shivering
- Reduced muscle tone or strength
- Abnormality of control of breathing
- Reduced tidal volume due to pain

Upper airway obstruction

It is always assumed that the commonest cause of upper airway obstruction is malpositioning of the head and neck before the patient is awake enough to maintain head position for themselves, allowing the root of the tongue to obstruct the pharynx or larynx. Fluoroscopic studies during sleep apnoea have rarely shown the tongue to be the main cause of obstruction. There is also fluoroscopic evidence that the soft palate is an important cause of obstructive episodes.[40] Even if the patient is in the semiprone "coma" position, upper airway obstruction can still occur.

Oedema, secretions, regurgitated stomach contents, blood, teeth or surgical debris may either cause an obstruction or may induce laryngeal spasm. If the mouth is closed the nasopharynx or nostrils may provide a high resistance to air flow, or may be completely blocked. If an artificial airway is still in place, this may be similarly blocked or kinked. Patients who are still under the influence of anaesthesia generally do not struggle against obstruction of the upper airway. Stridor, the noise of a partially obstructed upper airway, requires as urgent attention as complete obstruction: it is often a sign of laryngospasm, pharyngeal or laryngeal oedema, or epiglottic swelling. It must always be remembered that snoring is a form of upper respiratory tract obstruction.

Bronchospasm and functional residual capacity

Bronchospasm in the postoperative period may be due to pre-existing asthma, histamine release due to drug allergy, parasympathomimetic drugs, or response to foreign body inhalation, or it may be secondary to laryngospasm.

Functional residual capacity is reduced during anaesthesia because of a change in shape of the chest wall and a change in intrathoracic blood volume.[41]

Ventilation–perfusion imbalance

If a well perfused area of lung is poorly ventilated, gas exchange will be inefficient; this is called ventilation–perfusion imbalance or mismatch. Pre-existing disease, anaesthetics and abnormal position may cause an imbalance in the distribution of blood during the pulmonary circulation. Blood bypassing gas exchange in the lung is referred to as shunting.

Postoperative shivering

Shivering is a common postoperative occurrence; it is also known as halothane shakes, spontaneous postoperative tremor and pentothal shakes. The incidence is 5–65% in patients recovering from general anaesthesia, and shivering may also occur with spinal or epidural anaesthesia.[42] The incidence is higher in patients whose anaesthesia lasted for more than half an hour. The muscular activity of shivering causes a large increase in metabolic rate, with a consequent increase in oxygen consumption of as much as fivefold.[43] This occurs at a time when gas exchange may be compromised by other causes of postoperative hypoxaemia. It is therefore vital that oxygenation of the shivering patient is monitored carefully. This may be difficult, as shivering may cause failure of the pulse oximeter; it may cause artefactual erroneous indications of hypotension when non-invasive blood pressure measuring devices are used. There will be a concomitant rise in carbon dioxide production.

Reduced muscle tone or strength

Hypoventilation may be the result of reduced voluntary muscle tone and strength. This, in turn, may be due to abnormality in the function of the motor neurone, the neuromuscular junction, or the muscle cell itself.

Muscle tone is normally maintained by the gamma loop reflex, a feedback loop involving spindle stretch receptors in the muscle. Signals from these receptors travel to the spinal cord as sensory nerve fibres, activating anterior horn cells, which in turn stimulate the muscle fibres.

This simple loop system is controlled or modified by several factors. Those causing an increase in muscle tone are the central nervous system, circulating catecholamines, hypocalcaemia, alkalosis, tetanus and strychnine. Factors causing a decrease in muscle tone are hypoxia, hypotension and anaesthesia. Some of these modifying agents operate by way of the muscle cell or the peripheral nervous system, and some by both routes. Muscle weakness may be due to electrolyte imbalances, especially hypokalaemia, hypercalcaemia, hypophosphataemia, and generalised undernourishment or cachexia.

The commonest cause of respiratory muscle weakness in the recovery period is insufficient "reversal" of the pharmacological blockade of the neuromuscular junction. The state of the neuromuscular junction is best tested with a peripheral nerve stimulator. Possible abnormal findings include residual, unreversed competitive blockade; blockade owing to the use of suxamethonium in a patient with reduced levels of pseudocholinesterase; or a normally functioning neuromuscular junction with another cause for the weakness of the respiratory muscles. Enflurane, halothane and isoflurane all cause moderate skeletal muscle relaxation and enhance the effects of non-depolarising relaxants.

Abnormality of control of breathing

The respiratory control centres in the brain are greatly affected by anaesthetic agents, both intravenous and volatile, and also by opioids and sedative drugs. All will cause some degree of respiratory depression, ranging from clinically insignificant to respiratory arrest. Opioids are the drugs most likely to produce respiratory depression in the postoperative period; opioid analgesics induce a slow respiratory rate (bradypnoea) and diminished tidal volume. The normal hypoxic drive to ventilation is abolished by very low levels of volatile anaesthetic agents.[44]

Pain

Postoperative pain is a potent cause of hypoxaemia. Postoperative pain relief is important for both humanitarian and therapeutic reasons. Postoperative pain causes peripheral vasoconstriction, which may interfere with the function of a pulse oximeter, as may the concurrent restlessness. Pain reduces functional residual capacity, tidal volume and sputum clearance, and patients will also resist coughing. The normal event of sighing is also inhibited by pain and by sedative drugs. These effects all contribute to hypoxia, hypercapnia, atelectasis, ventilation–perfusion imbalance and shunting.

Postoperative pain relief, especially relief of abdominal or thoracic pain, increases oxygenation as tidal volume increases and active clearance of secretions becomes possible. In this case, giving opioids paradoxically causes a rise in arterial oxygen saturation. There is a much greater advantage in using local analgesia, as this will have no central depressive effect.

Transfer to the recovery room

Hypoxaemia occurring while a patient is being transferred from the operating table to the recovery room was rarely considered before the advent of pulse oximeter – this short period is often chaotic, and there was no satisfactory method of monitoring oxygen saturation while on the move. Monitoring 132 patients during transfer, Meiklejohn et al.[39] found that the oxygen saturation decreased to 85% or less in 22% of patients, and to 90% or less in 61·4%. They could identify no predictive factors, and the site of operation also had no bearing during this short period. They recommended that supplementary oxygen be given to all patients in the immediate postoperative period, including the period of transit to the recovery room.[39]

In the United States, Tyler et al.[45] found that during transfer hypoxaemia ($SpO_2 < 90\%$) occurred in 35% and severe hypoxaemia ($SpO_2 < 85\%$) in 12% of patients who had been breathing oxygen spontaneously before transfer. There was no correlation with age, anaesthetic agent, duration of anaesthesia or level of consciousness. There was a significant correlation between hypoxaemia and obesity. All the patients in the study who were mild asthma sufferers were in the severe hypoxia group.[45]

It is common practice to give 100% oxygen before taking patients off the operating table. This is done on the correct assumption that desaturation may occur owing to diffusion hypoxia. However, a few breaths of 100% oxygen before the patient is lifted are likely to maintain the blood fully oxygenated for only about 30 seconds, especially as ventilation is still likely to be depressed by anaesthetic agents, narcotics, and the residual effects of neurological blockade. The equilibration of PaO_2 or SpO_2 with inspired gas mixtures – in this case air – takes about 30 seconds even in normal volunteers.[46] Supplementary oxygen should therefore always be given during this period of transfer to the recovery room.

Early postoperative phase

The incidence of postoperative hypoxaemia in the recovery room has been well documented since the advent of the pulse oximeter.[47-53] There is, however, some discrepancy in the incidence, which ranges from 2% to 80% in different series. The difference might be explained if the saturation measurement were an instantaneous measurement made with a pulse oximeter or by continuous SpO_2 monitoring. Brown et al.[50] showed recently that postoperative hypoxaemia is often episodic, and thus intermittent measurements may well miss serious dips in saturation. Of 107 patients, 80% had at least one episode of $SpO_2 < 90\%$, and 26% of these had an $SpO_2 < 80\%$ during the first postoperative hour. However, when the same patients had discrete measurements of SpO_2 preoperatively and at five minutes and 30 minutes postoperatively, hypoxaemia was observed in 2%, 4% and 6% of patients at these times.[50]

Catley et al.[48] also found pronounced episodic oxygen desaturation in the postoperative period and investigated its association with ventilatory pattern and the method of analgesia used. They looked at two groups of 16 patients each recovering from general anaesthesia and major surgery. One group received a pain-relieving dose of morphine intravenously, followed by the same dose given continuously over the next 24 hours as an infusion. The other group received analgesia with bupivacaine. The patients were monitored over the first 16 hours. The two methods provided comparable analgesia, but there were quite different respiratory effects. Ten of the patients in the opioid group had a total of 456 episodes of pronounced desaturation, when the SpO_2 fell below 80%. These episodes all occurred while the patients were asleep and were all associated with ventilatory disturbances: obstructive apnoea, paradoxic breathing (with consequent very small tidal volume), and periods of bradypnoea. In contrast, the oxygen saturation of the patients receiving conduction analgesia never fell below 87%. The authors concluded that the interaction between sleep and opioid analgesia produced disturbances in ventilatory pattern, causing profound oxygen desaturation.[48]

Severe postoperative hypoxia may be predicted by one or more of the following risk factors: obesity (body mass index > 25), a body cavity procedure, age > 40 years, duration of surgery > 90 minutes, intravenous fluids > 1500 mL, and a combination of sleep and opioids (especially by infusion). Unrecognised hypoxaemia postoperatively is common with or without these risk factors, and therefore all patients should be monitored by pulse oximetry continuously for at least 45 minutes during this period.

The use of pulse oximetry in the recovery room is also of economic benefit, reducing the number of patients who require unexpected postoperative admission to the intensive care unit.[19]

Late postoperative hypoxaemia

Although it is common practice to give no less than 30% oxygen during anaesthesia and to give supplementary oxygen to patients in the recovery room, most patients revert to breathing air as soon as they return to the ward. It is the practice in many departments to give 40% oxygen for a further four hours after major surgery.

Of great concern should be recent reports of hypoxaemic episodes detected by pulse oximetry up to five days after major abdominal surgery.[18,41,54,55] Some of the factors influencing late postoperative hypoxaemia are listed in the Box.[18]

Factors associated with late postoperative hypoxaemia

Intrinsic
  Age and sex
  Pre-existing cardiovascular or respiratory disease
  Incision site and surgical procedure
  Sleep

Iatrogenic
  Pain and analgesics
  Anaesthetic technique
  Oxygen toxicity

Pulmonary complications
  Aspiration
  Atelectasis and infection
  Oedema
  Embolism

The commonest complication leading to late hypoxaemia was thought to be atelectasis. Although this is still an important reason, recent work suggests that episodic hypoxia is common for up to five days postoperatively.[54-56] Episodic desaturation is more likely to be due to the combination of opioids and sleep. Reeder *et al.*[54] continuously recorded oxygen saturation and electrocardiogram for 72 hours postoperatively. They noted a temporal relation between decreases in oxygen saturation and fluctuations in the ST segment level, indicating ischaemia. Episodic, and thus otherwise not noted without a pulse oximeter, desaturations may well be the cause of unexpected postoperative myocardial infarcts and arrhythmias. Reeder's group also monitored a number of patients before major surgery and then postoperatively for five consecutive nights. They found that oxygen supplementation was effective in keeping the saturation > 90% in the early postoperative period, but half the patients spent prolonged periods with an SpO_2 of < 85% during at least one night after operation. They concluded that oxygen supplementation should be considered beyond the usual clinical routine of one or two nights in patients who had undergone major abdominal surgery.[56]

Oxygen toxicity

During anaesthesia and throughout the postoperative phase, it is common practice – and indeed necessary – to give oxygen at greater concentrations than in the air. Though it may be felt that "if a little does you good, then more will do you better", it is well known that exposure to high concentrations of oxygen may be harmful. The rate at which oxygen toxicity develops is directly related to the partial pressure of inspired oxygen. The Apollo astronauts breathed 100% oxygen, apparently harmlessly, until the disastrous fire of 1967. The reason they showed no untoward toxicity was that the pressure in the capsule was only one-third of normal atmospheric pressure. For similar reasons, a high concentration of oxygen may be safely inspired at high altitude, in unpressurised aircraft and on mountains.

Symptoms of oxygen toxicity begin after an asymptomatic period of 6–12 hours. In conscious subjects, the symptoms and signs include tracheobronchial irritation (cough, substernal discomfort); tracheobronchitis; decreased clearance of mucus; decreased vital capacity; decreased pulmonary compliance; decreased diffusing capacity; increased arteriovenous shunting; and an increased ratio of dead space to tidal volume. Note that these occur in fit, healthy, young adults, who may tolerate hyperoxia for 24–48 hours without permanent pulmonary injury. The "safe" level of inspired oxygen is not established, but it is known that < 50% vol/vol can be tolerated for extended periods without deleterious effects.[57]

If high inspired oxygen pressures are maintained for > 36 hours in the fit volunteer, or for much shorter periods in the sick patient, pathological damage may occur. Lung hyperoxia leads to intracellular production of oxygen radicals, which in turn causes endothelial and epithelial damage and damage to lung macrophages. Chemotactic factors are released, leading to inflammation and further epithelial and endothelial destruction. There is impairment of the surfactant system, and pulmonary oedema is the final event before death.[57] It is thus important that enough oxygen is inspired in whatever situation to maintain oxygen saturation, but no more than is necessary.

9.4 Endoscopy

Endoscopy by way of any natural orifice is now a common and comparatively safe form of investigation. It yields as much, if not more, information than barium contrast radiological studies of the gastrointestinal tract, and includes the possibility of taking biopsies. Bronchoscopy has all but replaced contrast bronchography, and cystoscopy can now be undertaken in outpatients. These advances have been made possible by the flexible fibreoptic endoscope.

For most of these investigations, however, some form of sedation is usually given. The current sedative of choice is an intravenous benzodiazepine, usually midazolam. Midazolam given by this route is a powerful but fortunately short-acting hypnotic, anxiolytic and amnesic. The dose has to be large enough to sedate the patient but small enough to maintain their cooperation. Unfortunately, the endoscopy procedure always lasts for a much shorter time than the sedative effect of the drug. A further problem is that the surgeon or physician giving the sedative is usually also operating the endoscope. Although the sedation may be sufficient during the stimulation caused by the procedure, as soon as the stimulation ceases the patient often goes "deeper" during the recovery period and before the drug has been fully metabolised. A further danger to the oxygenation of the patient occurs during fibreoptic bronchoscopy, because of the instrumentation of the airway itself.

In view of the risk of hypoxaemia to the patient, the Endoscopy Committee working party of the British Society of Gastroenterology has published recommendations for the standard of sedation and patient monitoring during gastrointestinal endoscopy.[58] This recommends the use of pulse oximetry and that "clinical monitoring of the patient must be continued into the recovery area". I believe that all patients who are being sedated for any procedure should be monitored with pulse oximetry as a minimum.

It has been shown that complications of sedation are usually related to dysfunction of the cardiovascular system. Such complications are a manifestation of myocardial hypoxia and are therefore a function of arterial oxygen saturation. Unfortunately, without pulse oximetry, temporary cardiac hypoxia, which may cause permanent damage, often goes undetected. Shephard et al. have shown the relation between hypoxaemia, ventricular ectopics and sudden death.[59] Other workers have found that significant desaturation occurs during most endoscopic procedures under intravenous sedation.[60–64]

One of the most severe stresses on a patient in the endoscopy room is when undergoing endoscopic retrograde cholangiopancreatography (ERCP). The patient is normally in the prone position and sedated, and the procedure is relatively long. Harloff et al.[65] studied 75 patients undergoing the procedure and looked at age, weight, premedication, medical history, reason for examination, blood count, oxygen saturation, blood pressure, pulse, and length of procedure. Overall, there was considerable arterial desaturation in all patients; 32 patients (43%) had saturations < 90%, and two had episodes of SpO_2 < 70%.

There was no correlation with any of the preinvestigation findings. The authors advised that all patients undergoing ERCP should be monitored with pulse oximetry.[65]

Apart from the effects of sedation, the endoscope occupies a comparatively large cross-sectional area of the pharynx, increasing the resistance to flow of the respiratory gases. Furthermore, larger and larger instruments are being used for therapeutic procedures such as laser photocoagulation and electrodiathermy.[66]

Another severe stress on the patient is fibreoptic colonoscopy, which requires particularly heavy sedation. McKee *et al.* monitored 100 consecutive patients undergoing fibreoptic colonoscopy with a pulse oximeter. They found that 40 patients had SpO_2 < 90% after intravenous sedation but before colonoscopy; 14 patients had SpO_2 < 90% during colonoscopy; and 46 patients maintained SpO_2 > 90% throughout. They were unable to predict who would become hypoxic from age, body mass index, drug dose, or history of smoking, hypertension, diabetes, arrhythmias, or pulmonary or ischaemic heart disease. They concluded that all patients undergoing colonoscopy should be monitored with pulse oximetry and be given supplementary oxygen.[67]

Fibreoptic bronchoscopy

Patients undergoing fibreoptic bronchoscopy have three major features which militate against maintaining a normal level of arterial oxygen saturation: underlying pulmonary disease, "shared airway", and sedation for the procedure. The commonest reason for fibreoptic bronchoscopy is to elicit the cause of a mass found by chest radiography. If the mass causes symptoms then there is an increased likelihood that there is obstruction of a bronchial branch, and thus a ventilation–perfusion mismatch that already jeopardises oxygenation. Most patients with bronchial neoplasms also suffer from chronic obstructive pulmonary disease from the same cause: tobacco smoke. In these already compromised patients the fibreoptic bronchoscope decreases the cross-sectional area of the upper airways and increases the resistance to air flow. Furthermore, respiratory depression may be induced by sedative drugs. The sedation produced by, for example, short-acting benzodiazepines deepens immediately after the procedure, when the stimulation of the procedure ceases.

Maranetra *et al.* found a fall in SpO_2 of 1–25% (mean 5·6%) in 97 out of 100 consecutive patients undergoing diagnostic fibreoptic bronchoscopy. The recuperation time was 1–34 minutes (mean 8·2). The greatest aggravating factor was the patient being in the sitting position rather than supine; this was presumably due to ventilation–perfusion mismatch. The authors concluded that fibreoptic bronchoscopy should be carried out with the patient supine, with supplementary oxygen, and that a pulse oximeter be applied to every patient.[68] Pulse oximetry should also be continued into the recovery period.

Laser therapy

Although pulse oximetry should be used during all fibreoptic endoscopic procedures, there is a theoretical risk of the device overreading during and after the use of lasers or other forms of diathermy, in endoscopic surgery anywhere in the airway. This is due to the production of carbon monoxide by the burning tissue. This is absorbed and converts haemoglobin to carboxyhaemoglobin (see Chapter 11). The use of NdYAG lasers during bronchoscopy was investigated by Goldhill et al.,[69] who found that the mean preoperative carboxyhaemoglobin concentration of 1·4% was increased to a maximum of 2·05%. Many pulse oximeters are calibrated for a 1·4% carboxyhaemoglobin concentration, and therefore the rise to 2·05% produces an insignificant effect. Comparison of CO-oximetry with pulse oximetry showed a mean overread by the pulse oximeter of 1·03%. However, Goldhill et al'.s patients were being jet ventilated during the procedure, which may well have reduced the amount of carbon monoxide absorbed.

9.5 Dentistry and oral surgery

Although single-operator dental surgery under general anaesthesia is now no longer practised, many dental surgeons use some form of sedation, either inhalational or intravenous. A practitioner concentrating on the dental surgery cannot be expected to pay close attention to the state of oxygenation of the sedated patient. Likewise, the dental assistant cannot observe the patient continuously while carrying out his or her duties. Very few patients undergoing conscious sedation in the dental chair receive supplementary oxygen. It is common for non-anaesthetists to consider "sedation" as being harmless, especially when compared with general anaesthesia.

Hovagim et al. monitored 46 adult patients undergoing dental procedures with a pulse oximeter. Of these, 36 received some form of conscious sedation during the procedure, whereas 10 received only local anaesthesia; 28 patients received supplementary oxygen. In the control group there were only five episodes of mild hypoxaemia (3–5% below baseline saturation), whereas in the sedated group there were 316 episodes, 151 of which were mild, 132 moderate (6–10% below baseline saturation), and 33 severe (> 10% below baseline saturation). There was a significant correlation with a history of smoking, and also obesity. Hovagim *et al.* also found that, with the patients at risk, desaturation occurred despite supplementary oxygen.[70]

Tucker *et al.* compared the effects of different sedation regimens in outpatient dental surgery by looking at arterial oxygen tension, carbon dioxide tension, pH and oxygen saturation. They compared midazolam or diazepam, alone or in combination, with morphine or fentanyl given intravenously. They found much smaller falls in oxygen saturation than Hovagim's group, but the study may be criticised because the blood gas estimations were from discrete arterial samples taken infrequently; the oxygen saturations were presumably derived; whether supplementary oxygen was given was not mentioned; and the known periodic desaturations that occur with opioids were not taken into account.[71]

General anaesthesia

Many papers have recommended the use of pulse oximetry during general anaesthesia for dental procedures, pointing out that pulse oximeters should be applied to all patients even for short procedures; pulse oximetry alerts to desaturation before it is visible clinically; and pulse oximetry must continue until the patient has regained consciousness.[72–76] Significantly less desaturation occurs during the recovery phase if supplementary oxygen has been given, and if experienced recovery nurses are in attendance rather than locum staff.[75]

The expert working party

The Expert Working Party set up under Professor Poswillo to consider general anaesthesia, sedation and resuscitation in dentistry reported in 1990.[77] Among its principal recommendations are that a pulse oximeter is essential if general anaesthesia is to be given for dental procedures (paragraph 3.20). When patients are receiving sedation, "Dentists must be aware of the significance of pulse oximetry readings" (paragraph 4.15).

9.6 Sleep apnoea

There has been much interest in the investigation of sleep apnoea and other sleep disorders in recent years, especially since it has been possible to measure oxygenation non-invasively and cheaply with pulse oximeters. The recognition of the importance of sleep-related disorders is also recent, and it is related to work efficiency and safety. Reduction in sleep is associated with a decline in performance, especially with tasks that are repetitive or require high levels of vigilance.[78] Another important group of sleep disorders is those whose final common pathway is hypoxaemia; the results of this hypoxaemia include cerebrovascular accidents, cardiac arrhythmias and infarction, pulmonary hypertension, and right heart failure.

Main pathological problems associated with sleep disorders

- Insomnia
- Unpleasant dreams or nightmares
- Snoring
- Hypoxia
- Hypercapnia
- Somnolence

The functions of sleep are conservation of energy and restoration. The metabolic rate is reduced in sleep by 5–25%; restoration is thought to be both total body and neurological.[78] During sleep there is probably also increased protein synthesis and consolidation or enhancement of learning.[79]

Before discussing hypoxia during sleep disorders the organisation of sleep must be considered. The awake–asleep continuum has several stages.[80] Awake refers to the fully conscious state; drowsy is the transitional state between awake and asleep, and has also been referred to as wakefulness. There are two main types of sleep, REM (rapid eye movement) and non-REM. Non-REM sleep, also known as orthodox sleep, quiet sleep, and the S state, can be further categorised into four stages (Table 9.6.1).

During the awake but inactive state, the dominant influence on respiration is the metabolic state, which is mediated by chemoreceptors. This control is overridden during talking, laughing, coughing, and also during vomiting, or when conscious control of breathing is assumed. During non-REM sleep breathing is under control of the metabolic state. During REM sleep, however, although the metabolic state predominates in the control of respiration, any

Table 9.6.1 The stages of sleep. Reproduced by permission of J Kagan and J Segal and Harcourt, Brace, Jovanovitch[81]

Stage	EEG	Behaviour or sensations	Depth of sleep	Physiological changes	Dreams	Control of respiration
Non-REM 1	Low amplitude; mixed frequency; no sleep spindles; no K complexes	Sometimes a floating sensation; drifting with idle thoughts and dreams	Can still be easily awakened and will insist has not been asleep	Muscles relaxing; pulse becomes even; breathing becomes regular; temperature falling	Images and thought-like fragments	Metabolic
Non-REM 2	Low amplitude, growing larger; mixed frequency; bursts of high amplitude and low frequency: sleep spindles	If eyes are open, will not see	May be awakened with a modest sound	Eyes roll slowly from side to side	Some thought-like fragments and low intensity dreams	Metabolic
Non-REM 3	20–50% higher amplitude, lower frequency	Removed from conscious world	Takes louder noise to awaken	Muscles relaxed; breathing even; heart rate slowed; temperature slightly down; muscle tone reduced; blood pressure reduced	Rarely recalled	Metabolic
Non-REM 4	High amplitude, low frequency for > 50%; sleep spindles may be present	May begin sleep walking or bed wetting	The deepest sleep; most difficult to awaken	Even breathing; even heart rate; even blood pressure; temperature slowly reduces	Poor recall makes this seem a dreamless oblivion most of the time; rare nightmares	Metabolic
REM	Low amplitude, mixed frequency; saw-toothed waves may occur	Rapid eye movements (REMs) as if watching something	Hard to bring to consciousness and reality	Muscle tone reduced; penile erection; increased vaginal congestion; increased gastrointestinal secretions; labile blood pressure; heart rate irregular; respiration irregular	Very vivid dreams 85% of time	?Behavioural
						Metabolic

Kagan J, Segal J, 1988, *Psychology – an introduction* published by Harcourt, Brace, Jovanovitch, Orlando, USA, page 325.

rapid changes in the metabolic state are thought to have a decreased effect on respiration; this is of little importance, as REM sleep occurs in short episodes.[82]

Hypoxia during sleep

The commonest cause of hypoxia during sleep is episodic apnoea. There are two main subdivisions of sleep apnoea, central and obstructive. Central sleep apnoea is comparatively rare compared with obstructive causes.[83] The overall incidence of the sleep apnoeas is 1–3% with a male predominance.[84]

Clinical distinguishing features of central and obstructive sleep apnoea

Central	Obstructive
Very rare (10%)	Common (90%)
Insomnia	Patient is often obese
Hypersomnolence is rare	Daytime hypersomnolence
Often awake during sleep	Rarely awake during sleep
Occasional mild snoring	Loud snoring
Depression	Intellectual deterioration
No airway obstruction	Sexual dysfunction
	Morning headache
	Nocturia

The most important difference between central and obstructive apnoea is that there is no obstructive element in the central type. However, most workers consider that in many cases there is a mixture of central and obstructive types. The evidence for this lies in studies of patients who have had a tracheostomy to relieve obstructive sleep apnoea. Most of these patients show evidence of central apnoea for some months, after which apnoea slowly resolves.[85]

Central sleep apnoea

During wakefulness, the control of the respiratory muscles by way of the respiratory centre in the brain stem comes from three sources: "waking neural drive"; the behavioural control system, which is concerned with activities such as speaking; and the metabolic control system, which has inputs from chemoreceptors (oxygen, carbon dioxide, and hydrogen ions) and vagal afferents. During sleep, the waking neural drive and the behavioural control are lost. The underlying mechanisms of central sleep apnoea may be one of those shown in the Box.[86]

Underlying mechanisms of central sleep apnoea

Defects in the metabolic control system:
  Primary or secondary central alveolar hypoventilation

Respiratory muscle weakness:
  Transient instability in the central drive mechanism
  Sleep onset
  Hypocapnia induced by hyperventilation
  Prolonged circulation time

Reflex inhibition of central respiratory drive:
  Upper airway collapse
  Oesophageal reflux
  Aspiration of secretions or stomach contents

Before considering treatment of central sleep apnoea, it is necessary further to subdivide apparent sufferers according to whether or not they are hypercapnic. The hypercapnic group have hypoxaemic episodes at night, and pulse oximetry recordings form an essential part of the diagnostic evidence. The non-hypercapnic group have relatively mild arterial desaturation; although they also have hypoxaemic episodes, these are less severe and are usually around the flat horizontal part of the oxyhaemoglobin dissociation curve.[87]

Obstructive sleep apnoea

Obstructive sleep apnoea is one of the commonest causes of arterial oxygen desaturation during sleep. As it often causes snoring or other stridulous noises, it is often looked on with mirth and is the subject of many humorous anecdotes. Obstructive sleep apnoea is not a separate entity from snoring but an extreme part of a continuum of upper airway obstruction that ranges from very mild to severe. Obstructive sleep apnoea is important as there is growing evidence of secondary effects, which were originally thought to be idiopathic. The effects on the cardiovascular system may be particularly dramatic.

Patients with obstructive sleep apnoea are considered to be at increased risk of sudden death during sleep, presumably related to arrhythmia. Shepard *et al.*[88] reported a strong relationship between obstructive sleep apnoea and ventricular ectopic beats. They looked at 31 male patients with obstructive sleep apnoea. Recordings were made of oxygen saturation, electrocardiographic variables, respiratory air flow (with thermistors), and thoracoabdominal movement (by thoracic impedance pneumonography) during sleep. Premature ventricular complexes were found in 23% of the subjects. Ventricular bigeminy was recorded in 16 of the subjects and was associated with desaturation to below 60%.[88] Deedwania et al.[89] found nocturnal atrioventricular conduction block as a manifestation of desaturation during sleep apnoea. Saito et al.,[90] using pulse oximetry, electrocardiography and an apnoea monitor, reported myocardial infarction complicating sleep apnoea. Sustained episodes of hypoxaemia may lead to pulmonary vasoconstriction, pulmonary hypertension, and eventually right-sided heart failure.[91,92]

The incidence of cerebrovascular accidents or strokes is reported to be higher in those who are snorers or are known to have obstructive sleep apnoea.[93] The mechanisms by which snoring or obstructive sleep apnoea may increase the incidence of strokes may include cyclical increases in intracranial pressure that coincide with increases in systemic blood pressure; these increases are associated with episodes of desaturation and normally occur during REM sleep. Impaired intracranial autoregulation also contributes to the aetiology.

Other sequelae of obstructive sleep apnoea include polycythaemia, abnormal motor activity during sleep, morning headache, intellectual deterioration, hypnogogic hallucinations, automatic behaviour, short-term memory loss, personality changes, sexual impotence and nocturnal enuresis.

Anatomy and physiology of obstructive sleep apnoea

Figure 9.6.1 summarises the anatomical factors in obstructive sleep apnoea. Various imaging techniques may be used to investigate the upper airways (Box).

Factors contributing to upper airway obstruction during sleep[94,95]

- Anatomical narrowing of the upper airway
- Increased compliance or collapsability of upper airway tissues
- Reflexes acting on upper airway calibre
- Pharyngeal inspiratory muscle function

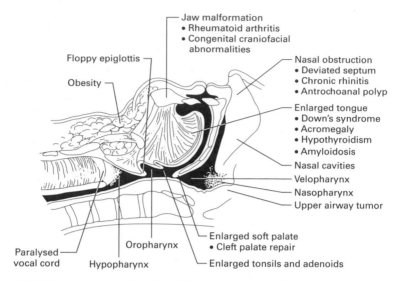

Figure 9.6.1 Upper airway, showing different segments of pharynx and various abnormalities reported to cause obstructive sleep apnoea. Reproduced with permission.[96]

Imaging techniques for investigation of upper airway

- Cephalometry (plain radiograms)
- Computed tomography
- Fluoroscopy
- Magnetic resonance imaging
- Direct nasopharyngoscopy
- Acoustic reflection studies

Of these investigations, the only unusual one is acoustic reflection. At present this is used only in research. The technique is based on the reflection of incident soundwaves in the airways. A major advantage of the technique is that studies can be made every 200 ms. Figure 9.6.2 (from Rivlin *et al.*[97]) shows an acoustic reflection area–distance plot for a normal subject and a patient with obstructive sleep apnoea and clearly shows a reduction in the cross-sectional area of the patient's airway.

Computed tomography of the pharynx, taken with the patient awake and then sleeping, shows the lateral pharyngeal walls folding inward, along with a retrodisplacement of the tongue, thereby demonstrating the circumferential nature of the airway collapse during sleep.[98]

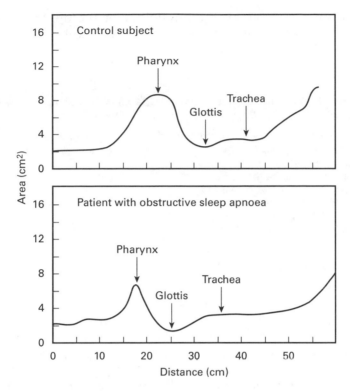

Figure 9.6.2 Acoustic reflection area–distance function for control subject and patient with obstructive sleep apnoea; anatomical landmarks are identified. Reproduced with permission.[97]

Hereditary and acquired anatomical variations that may precipitate obstructive sleep apnoea are listed in the Box.[94,95]

Anatomical abnormalities associated with obstructive sleep apnoea

- Adenoid and tonsillar hypertrophy
- Glottal web
- Vocal cord paralysis
- Acromegaly
- Lymphoma or Hodgkin's disease in pharyngeal lymphoid tissue
- Micrognathia, retrognathia
- Ectopic thyroid, thyroid hypertrophy
- Upper airway oedema or fibrosis
- Severe kyphoscoliosis
- Corrected velopharyngeal incompetence in infants
- Cushing's disease or syndrome

Pathological alterations in the physiology of the upper airway also occur in obstructive sleep apnoea; these have also been summarised by Hudgel (Box).[94,95]

Physiological abnormalities predisposing to obstructive sleep apnoea

- Poliomyelitis, muscular dystrophy, motor neurone disease, and other diseases with bulbar incoordination secondary to brainstem abnormalities
- Acquired dysautonomia
- Diaphragm pacing for primary alveolar hypoventilation
- Hypothyroidism
- Drug-induced sedation
- Alcohol ingestion
- Treatment with testosterone
- Epilepsy
- Encephalitis

Pulse oximetry with continuous recording during sleep is an important test in the assessment of obstructive sleep apnoea, especially if surgical treatment is being contemplated. The use of pulse oximetry as a screening test for sleep apnoea has been validated by Cooper *et al.*[99] who compared pulse oximetry with a polysonographic package that included measurement of chest wall movement with magnetometers and of air flow at the nose and mouth with thermocouples, and an electroencephalogram and electro-oculogram. Overnight pulse oximetry was found to be highly specific as an initial screening test for sleep apnoea.[99]

In an attempt to simplify the assessment of sleep apnoea/hypopnoea syndrome (SAHS), the British Thoracic Society found that patients with more than 15·4% desaturations per hour of < 90% SpO_2 all proved to suffer from the syndrome. However, this test, although highly specific, may miss patients with SAHS who have hypopnoeic episodes which cause arousal but not significant desaturation.[100] Awake SpO_2 is a very poor predictor of noctural oxygen desaturation.[101]

The treatment of obstructive sleep apnoea depends on the severity of symptoms, the aetiology of the obstruction, and the risk of complications of obstructive sleep apnoea in a particular patient. Common treatments are shown in the Box.[94,95] Pulse oximetry should be repeated after any surgical treatment to measure the efficacy of the treatment.

Treatments for obstructive sleep apnoea

- Weight reduction
- Relief of nasal obstruction
- Avoidance of alcohol in the evening
- Nasal continuous positive airway pressure (CPAP)
- Uvulopalatopharyngoplasty
- Maxillomandibular surgery
- Intraoral appliance

Obstructive sleep apnoea in children

By far the commonest cause of obstructive sleep apnoea in paediatric practice is hyperplasia of the tonsils and adenoids.[102] There is convincing evidence that children who snore have nocturnal hypoxaemia, together with abnormal sleep patterns and a higher incidence of hyperactivity, daytime somnolence, aggression and learning difficulties.

Before the introduction of pulse oximetry, objective investigation of suspicions of sleep apnoea in children required expensive multi-parameter polysomnography (respiratory air flow, chest wall movement, electroencephalogram, electro-oculogram).[103] Stradling et al. looked at a series of 61 snoring children between the ages of 2 and 14 years selected for tonsillectomy, mainly for recurrent tonsillitis. Preoperative, overnight continuous pulse oximetry, among other variables, showed a much higher and more frequent incidence of hypoxaemic episodes in snorers than in normal matched control children. Recordings made six months after adenotonsillectomy showed an appreciable reduction in hypoxaemic episodes, equivalent to the controls. Sleep disturbances and multiple other symptoms resolved, and a growth spurt occurred.[104]

Postic et al.[102] found certain common manifestations in the history of children with adenotonsillar hyperplasia and obstructive sleep apnoea. Snoring, breath holding, night cough and nocturnal enuresis were related to sleep; in the daytime the children experienced morning irascibility, mouth breathing, slow eating, dry mouth, trouble swallowing, and daytime fatigue.[102] Pulse oximetry is an easy and economical method of assessing the severity of obstructive sleep apnoea in children presenting with these symptoms.

Patients with chronic obstructive airways disease usually become hypoxic during sleep, particularly during REM sleep. This may be due to hypoventilation, decrease in functional residual capacity, ventilation–perfusion mismatching or sleep apnoea.[105]

Nocturnal asthma

Many patients find that their asthma is worse at night, with broncho-constriction often at its worst on waking; these patients are sometimes referred to as morning dippers. During these dips hypoxaemia is often detected by pulse oximetry, although in otherwise healthy asthmatic patients the lowest saturation is in the range 95–85%.[106] Catterall *et al.* found no correlation between the extent of hypoxaemia and the degree of overnight bronchoconstriction in adults, the extent of desaturation being more predictable from the level of saturation during waking.[107] Smith and Hudgel,[108] however, found that nocturnal hypoxaemia in asthmatic children correlated well with the overnight fall in forced expiratory volume.

9.7   Neonatal pulse oximetry

Pulse oximetry is becoming a common technique for assessing arterial oxygenation in neonates. Continuous online indication of the oxygenation of the sick neonate is needed. Two decades ago such continuous monitoring was not possible and discrete blood gas analysis was necessary, either from capillary samples or from arterial samples in very sick ventilated patients. This was superseded by transcutaneous blood gas analysis, in which miniature Clarke (PO_2) and Severinghaus (PCO_2) electrodes are applied to the skin. The electrodes contain heaters to "arterialise" the capillary blood flow. The pulse oximeter is compared with the transcutaneous oxygen tension monitor in the Box.

The first consideration in the use of pulse oximeters on neonates must be that the device is calibrated for human adult haemoglobin, HbA. The extinction coefficients for the wavelengths currently used in pulse oximetry are virtually identical for HbA and for fetal haemoglobin, HbF.[109,110] Nijland *et al.*[111] reinforce the point that pulse oximeters are calibrated for HbA between about 75% and 100% saturation. They found that pulse oximeters calibrated for adults underestimate arterial oxygen saturation at very low levels – around 25%, a value that may occur in a fetus during labour. There has been some confusion in the literature over this point, as oxygen saturation often differs between pulse oximetry and discrete sample CO-oximetry.[110] This is because the two techniques measure saturation over different ranges of wavelength: whereas the absorption spectra are virtually identical over the range used in pulse oximetry, there are differences in the wavelengths used in CO-oximetry.[112-114] Because of the range of wavelengths used, pulse oximetry may be assumed to be a safe technique to use with neonates.

Pulse oximetry, rather than transcutaneous blood gas analysis, is increasingly popular because of its low capital cost, low running cost, ease of application and low morbidity, and because no calibration is required. It must be remembered, however, that the two techniques measure different things. Pulse oximetry gives an approximation of arterial haemoglobin oxygen saturation, whereas transcutaneous blood gas analysis gives an approximation of the partial pressure of oxygen in the plasma of "arterialised" capillaries. As pointed out in Chapter 6, these are two different measurements and the results obtained are not directly interchangeable.

Assessing arterial oxygenation in neonates

Pulse oximeter	Transcutaneous oxygen tension monitor
Advantages	
Continuous SaO_2 (SpO_2)	Continuous PaO_2 (transcutaneous PaO_2)
Multiple choices of site	Non-invasive
No warm-up time	Functions with failing
Non-invasive	cardiovascular system
Direct reading of signal strength	
Tissue injury unlikely	
No calibration required	
Easy application sensor	
Indication of cardiac rhythm	
Negligible running cost	
Multiple monitoring sites available	
Wide variety of sensor	
configurations	
"Accurate" reading or no	
reading at all	
Disadvantages	
Affected by ambient light	Correlation with PaO_2 reduced by
May be affected by pulsatile veins	low blood flow
No trend until $PaO_2 < 70$ mmHg	No indication of signal strength
Calibration not available	Long warm up time
RF diathermy causes errors	Thermal injury common
Motion artefacts	Requires membrane changes
Pulsatile signal needed	Requires frequent calibration
May fail in anaemia	Requires frequent site changes
May be affected by dyes	Sensor application not easy
Does not indicate PaO_2	Expensive to purchase and use

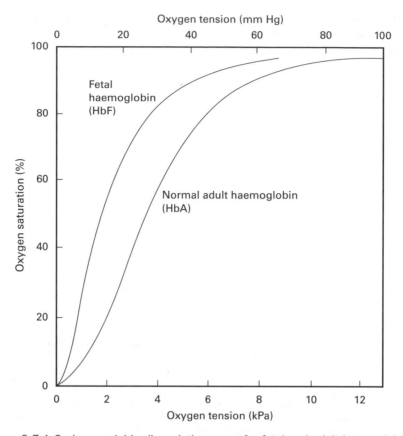

Figure 9.7.1 Oxyhaemoglobin dissociation curve for fetal and adult haemoglobin.

Figure 9.7.1 compares the oxyhaemoglobin dissociation curve for fetal haemoglobin with that for adult haemoglobin. As in adults, a number of factors may cause a shift in the curve, and many of these factors may cause the curve to shift much more rapidly in infants than in adults.

The great concern of neonatal paediatricians is to prevent retinopathy of prematurity, formerly known as retrolental fibroplasia. Retinopathy of prematurity may cause blindness in premature babies of less than 28 weeks' gestation and birthweight of less than 1500 g; it is unusual in babies of over 32 weeks' gestation. High levels of retinal oxygenation are thought to cause spasm of the developing vasculature, leading to ischaemia. This is possible with arterial oxygen partial pressure over 20 kPa or 150 mmHg.[115] Several authors state that the SpO_2 should be kept "below 95%: 80%–90% is safe";[116] < 95% ("PaO_2 > 90 mmHg")is safe;[117] > 92% "may be associated with

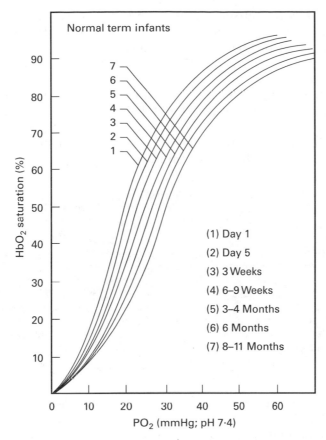

Figure 9.7.2 Oxyhaemoglobin dissociation curves of infants of different ages; curves represent mean values. Reproduced with permission.[121]

hyperoxia";[118] 80%–95% is safe;[119] "a limit of 93% is likely to maintain PaO$_2$ below 12 kPa."[121] However, many authors fail to take into account that SpO$_2$ often correlates poorly with the partial pressure of oxygen in the plasma, as so many factors may cause a shift in the neonate's oxyhaemoglobin dissociation curve (see box on p 132).

A further factor that causes a shift in the oxyhaemoglobin dissociation curve of the neonate is the slow decrease in the concentration of fetal haemoglobin and increase in adult haemoglobin (Figure 9.7.2). In the worst case, an SpO$_2$ of 80% may correspond to a PaO$_2$ of about 30 mmHg, with consequent hypoxic damage.

It is often difficult to apply the pulse oximeter probe to very small fingers or ears. This may lead to malfunction; in most cases the malfunction causes an alarm condition, but often the device will indicate a falsely low SpO$_2$. This is caused by what has been termed the penumbra effect[122] and is due to the red and infrared light-emitting diodes not being exactly mechanically incident with each other. On an adult patient a difference in axis of 1–3 mm is unlikely to cause a problem, but with very small fingers there may be a comparatively large difference in path length between each diode and the detector. Thus one of the channels is grossly overloaded, causing an erroneous result. An unexpectedly low reading may suddenly improve if the probe is repositioned. Most of the larger manufacturers make special probes for small children.

Causes of displacement of oxyhaemoglobin dissociation curve

Left displacement	*Right displacement*
Decrease in hydrogen ion concentration	Increase in hydrogen ion concentration
Decrease in temperature	Increase in temperature
Decrease in PCO$_2$	Increase in PCO$_2$
Decrease in 2,3-DPG in red blood cells	Increase in 2,3-DPG
Decrease in ATP in red blood cells	Increase in ATP in red blood cells
Increase in carboxyhaemoglobin	Decrease in zinc in red blood cells
Increase in methaemoglobin	Abnormal haemoglobins
Abnormal haemoglobins	

There have been several reports of "burns" caused by pulse oximetry on small children. It is most unlikely that these are actually burns caused by heat energy from the light-emitting diodes and much more likely that they are caused by pressure necrosis, due either to the probe being applied too tightly or to poor perfusion of the skin under the probe.[123,124] It is important that probes are not applied too tightly; most neonatal probes are attached with Velcro or adhesive tape. Burns under the probe are theoretically possible when radiofrequency diathermy is in use, but good electrical design should reduce this risk.

Low SpO$_2$ readings in small children may also be caused by increased pulsatility of venules owing to the short length of the capillaries.

Pulse oximetry should also form part of the multichannel polysomnographic recordings for the evaluation of apnoea in infants. These investigations may form part of the investigations for the risk of sudden infant death syndrome. Pulse oximetry with recordings made for 24 hours should be part of the routine management of all high-risk neonates and infants with respiratory or cardiorespiratory problems,[125] and especially when investigating cyanotic apnoeic attacks, laryngomalacia and other causes of obstructive sleep apnoea.

In summary, in neonates and infants pulse oximetry is as safe as in adults, with less morbidity than transcutaneous oxygen monitoring, as long as the oxyhaemoglobin dissociation curve is taken into account, the probe is positioned properly, and care is taken with the fixing of the probe.

Plethysmography using a pulse oximeter[126] and a cuff has been shown to be a more accurate method of measuring neonatal arterial blood pressure non-invasively than the oscillometric method.

References

1 Anderson ID, Woodford M, de Dombal FT, Irving M. Retrospective study of 1000 deaths from injury in England and Wales. *BMJ* 1988;**296**:1305–8.
2 Comroe JH, Botelho S. The unreliability of cyanosis in the recognition of arterial anoxemia. *Am J Med Sci* 1947;**214**:1–6.
3 Brown LH, Manring EA, Kornegay HB, Prasad NH. Can pre-hospital personnel detect hypoxemia without the aid of a pulse oximeter? *Am J Emerg Med* 1996;**14**:43–4.
4 Cockroft S, Dodd P. Pulse oximetry at the roadside. *BMJ* 1989;**298**:1096.
5 Moyle JTB. Pulse oximetry at the roadside. *BMJ* 1989;**298**:1096.
6 Silverstone P. Pulse oximetry at the roadside: a study of pulse oximetry in immediate care. *BMJ* 1989;**298**:711–3.
7 Craft TM, Blogg CE. Pulse oximetry at the roadside. *BMJ* 1989;**298**:1096.
8 McGuire TJ, Pointer JE. Evaluation of a pulse oximeter in the prehospital setting. *Ann Emerg Med* 1988;**17**:1058–62.
9 Aughey K, Hess D, Eitel D *et al*. An evaluation of pulse oximetry in prehospital care. *Ann Emerg Med* 1991;**20**:877–91.
10 Bota G, Rowe G. Pulse oximetry study: does unrecognised hypoxia exist in the prehospital setting? *Ann Emerg Med* 1992;**21**:479.
11 Maneker AJ, Petrack EM, Krug SE. Contribution of routine pulse oximetry to evaluation and management of patients with respiratory illness in a pediatric emergency department. *Ann Emerg Med* 1995;**25**:36–40.
12 Mower WR, Sachs C, Nicklin EL, Baraff LJ. Pulse oximetry as a fifth pediatric vital sign. *Pediatrics* 1997;**99**:681–6.
13 Wright SW. Conscious sedation in the emergency department: value of capnography and pulse oximetry. *Ann Emerg Med* 1992;**21**:551–5.
14 Lambert MA, Crinnion J. The role of pulse oximetry in the accident and emergency department. *Arch Emerg Med* 1989;**6**:211–15.
15 David HG. Pulse oximetry in closed limb fractures. *Ann Roy Coll Surg Eng* 1991;**73**:283–4.
16 Kellerman AL, Cofer CA, Joseph S, Hackman BB. *Ann Emerg Med* 1991;**20**:130–4.
17 Comroe JH, Botelho S. The unreliability of cyanosis in the recognition of arterial hypoxemia. *Am J Med Sci* 1947;**214**:1–6.
18 Marshall BE, Wyche MQ. Hypoxemia during and after anesthesia. *Anesthesiology* 1972;**37**:178–208.

19 Brodsky JB, McKilveen RE, Zelcer J, Margary JJ. Diffusion hypoxia: a reappraisal using pulse oximetry. *J Clin Monit* 1988;**4**:244–6.

20 Heneghan CPH, Bergman NA, Jones JG. Changes in lung volume and (PAO_2–PAO_2) during anaesthesia. *Br J Anaesth* 1984;**56**:437–45.

21 Moller JT, Johannessen NW, Berg H, Espersen K, Larsen LE. Hypoxaemia during anaesthesia – an observer study. *Br J Anaesth* 1991;**66**:437–44.

22 Moller JT, Jensen PF, Johannessen NW, Espersen K. Hypoxaemia is reduced by pulse oximetry monitoring in the operating theatre and in the recovery room. *Br J Anaesth* 1992;**68**:146–50.

23 Drummond GB, Park GR. Arterial oxygen saturation before intubation of the trachea. *Br J Anaesth* 1984;**56**:987–92.

24 Benumof JL, Dagg R, Benumof R. Critical hemoglobin desaturation will occur before return to an unparalyzed state following 1 mg/kg intravenous succinylcholine. *Anesthesiology* 1997;**87**:979–82.

25 Kong AS, Brennan L, Bingham R, Morgan-Hughes J. An audit of anaesthesia in neonates and small infants using pulse oximetry. *Anaesthesia* 1992;**47**:896–9.

26 Duberman SM, Bendixen HH. Concepts of fail-safe anesthetic practice. *Int Anesthesiol Clin* 1989;**22**:149–65.

27 Peterson AW, Jacken LM. Death following inadvertent esophageal intubation: a case report. *Anesth Analg* 1973;**52**:398–401.

28 Guggenberger H, Lenz G, Federle R. Early detection of inadvertent oesophageal intubation: pulse oximetry vs capnography. *Acta Anaesthesiol* 1989;**33**:112–5.

29 Sosis MB, Sisamis J. Pulse oximetry in confirmation of correct tracheal tube placement. *Anesth Analg* 1990;**71**:305–14.

30 Barker SJ, Tremper KK, Hyatt J, Heitzmann H. Comparison of three oxygen monitors in detecting endobronchial intubation. *J Clin Monit* 1988;**4**:240–3.

31 Haynes SR, Allsop JR, Gillies GWA. Arterial oxygen saturation during induction of anaesthesia and laryngeal mask insertion: prospective evaluation of four techniques. *Br J Anaesth* 1992;**68**:519–22.

32 Wilkins CJ, Moores M, Hanning CD. Comparison of pulse oximeters: effects of vasoconstriction and venous engorgement. *Br J Anaesth* 1989;**62**:439–44.

33 Verhoeff F, Sykes MK. Delayed detection of hypoxic events by pulse oximeters: computer simulations. *Anaesthesia* 1990;**45**:103–9.

34 Gruber P, Kwaitkowski T, Silverman R, Flaster E, Auerbch C. Time to equilibration of oxygen saturation using pulse oximetry. *Acad Emerg Med* 1995;**2**:810–14.

35 Cook RI, Block FE, McDonald JS. Cascade of monitor detection of anesthetic disaster. *Anesthesiology* 1988;**69**:A277.

36 Smith DC, Crul JF. Oxygen desaturation following sedation for regional analgesia. *Br J Anaesth* 1989;**62**:206–9.

37 Mineo R, Sharrock NE. Pulse oximeter waveforms from the finger and toe during lumbar epidural anesthesia. *Regional Anesth* 1993;**18**:106–9.

38 Nunn JF, Payne JP. Hypoxaemia after general anaesthesia. *Lancet* 1962;**ii**:631–2.

39 Meiklejohn BH, Smith G, Elling AE, Hindocha N. Arterial oxygen desaturation during postoperative transportation: the influence of operation site. *Anaesthesia* 1987;**42**:1313–15.

40 Rodenstein DO, Stanescu DC. The soft palate and breathing. *Am Rev Respir Dis* 1986;**134**:311–25.

41 Jones JG, Sapsford DJ, Wheatley RG. Postoperative hypoxaemia: mechanisms and time course. *Anaesthesia* 1990;**45**:566–73.

42 Crossley AWA. Postoperative shivering. *Br J Hosp Med* 1993;**49**:204–8.

43 MacIntyre PE, Pavlin EG, Dwersteg JF. Effect of meperidine on oxygen consumption, carbon dioxide production and respiratory gas exchange in postanesthesia shivering. *Anesth Analg* 1987:751–5.

44 Knill RL, Gelb AW. Ventilatory responses to hypoxia and hypercapnia during holothane sedation and anaesthesia in man. *Anesthesiology* 1978;**49**:244–51.

45 Tyler IL, Tantisira B, Winter PM. Continuous monitoring of arterial oxygen saturation with pulse oximetry during transfer to the recovery room. *Anesth Analg* 1985;**64**:1108–12.

46 Ernsting J. The effect of brief profound hypoxia upon arterial and venous tensions in man. *J Physiol* 1963;**169**:292–311.

47 Canet J, Ricos M, Vidal F. Early postoperative arterial oxygen desaturation: determining factors and response to oxygen therapy. *Anesth Analg* 1989;**69**:207–12.

48 Catley DM, Thornton C, Jordan C, Lehane JR, Royston D, Jones JG. Pronounced episodic oxygen desaturation in the postoperative period: its association with ventilatory pattern and analgesic regimen. *Anesthesiology* 1985;**63**:20–8.

49 Lehmann KA, Asoklis S, Grond S, Huttarsch H. [Development of a method of continuous monitoring or spontaneous respiration in the postoperative phase.] *Anaesthesist* 1992;**41**:121–9. (In German; English abstract.)

50 Brown LT, Purcell GJ, Traugott FM. Hypoxaemia during postoperative recovery using continuous pulse oximetry. *Anaesth Intensive Care* 1990;**18**:509–16.

51 Morris RW, Buschman A, Philip JH, Raemer DB. The prevalence of hypoxaemia, detected by pulse oximetry during recovery from anaesthesia. *J Clin Monit* 1988;**4**:16–20.

52 Laycock GJA, McNicol LR. Hypoacmia during recovery from anaesthesia—an audit of children after general anaesthesia for routine elective surgery. *Anaesthesia* 1988;**43**:984–7.

53 Smith DC, Canning JJ, Crul JF. Pulse oximetry in the recovery room. *Anaesthesia* 1989;**44**:345–8.

54 Reeder MK, Muir AD, Foex P, Goldman MD, Loh L, Smart D. Postoperative myocardial ischaemia: temporal association with nocturnal hypoxaemia. *Br J Anaesth* 1991;**67**:626–31.

55 Rosenberg J, Rasmussen V, von Jessen F, Ulstad T, Kehlet H. Late postoperative episodic and constant hypoxaemia and associated ECG abnormalities. *Br J Anaesth* 1990;**65**:684–91.

56 Reeder MK, Goldman MD, Loh L *et al*. Postoperative hypoxaemia after major abdominal vascular surgery. *Br J Anaesth* 1991;**68**:23–6.

57 Klein J. Oxygen toxicity–review article. *Anesth Analg* 1990;**70**:195–207.
58 Bell GD, McCloy RF, Charlton JE *et al*. Recommendations for standards of sedation and monitoring during gastrointestinal endoscopy. *Gut* 1991;**32**:823–7.
59 Shephard JW, Garrison MW, Grither DA, Evans R, Schweitzer PK. Relationship of ventricular ectopy to nocturnal oxygen desaturation in patients with chronic obstructive pulmonary disease. *Am J Med* 1985;**78**:28–34.
60 Hayward SR, Sugawa C, Wilson RF. Changes in oxygenation and pulse rate during endoscopy. *Am Surg* 1989;**55**:198–202.
61 Visco DM, Tolpin E, Straughn JC, Fagraeus L. Arterial oxygen saturation in sedated patients undergoing gastrointestinal endoscopy and a review of pulse oximetry. *Del Med J* 1989;**61**:533–42.
62 Bailey PL, Pace NL, Ashburn MA, Moll JW, East KA, Stanley TH. Frequent hypoxaemia and apnea after sedation with midazolam and fentanyl. *Anaesthesiology* 1990;**73**:826–30.
63 Schnapf BM. Oxygen desaturation during fibreoptic bronchoscopy in pediatric patients. *Chest* 1991;**99**:591–4.
64 Murray AW, Morran CG, Kenny GNC, Anderson JR. Arterial oxygen saturation during upper gastrointestinal endoscopy: the effects of a midazolam/pethidine combination. *Gut* 1990;**31**:270–3.
65 Harloff M, Weber J, Kohler B, Astheimer W, Wagner M, Rieman JF. [Importance of cardiocirculatory and pulmonary monitoring in endoscopic retrograde cholangiopancreatography]. *Z Gastroenterol* 1991;**29**:387–91. (In German.)
66 Bell GD, Morden A, Bown S, Coady T, Logan RFA. Prevention of hypoxaemia during upper gastrointestinal endoscopy by means of oxygen via nasal cannulae. *Lancet* 1987;**i**:1022–3.
67 McKee CC, Ragland JJ, Myers JO. An evaluation of multiple clinical variables for hypoxia during colonoscopy. *Surg Gynecol Obstet* 1991;**173**:37–40.
68 Maranetra N, Pushakum R, Bovornkitti S. Oxygen desaturation during fibreoptic bronchoscopy. *J Med Assoc Thai* 1990;**73**:258–63.
69 Goldhill DR, Hill AJ, Whitburn RH, Feneck RO, George PJ, Keeling P. Carboxyhaemoglobin concentrations, pulse oximetry and arterial blood-gas tensions during jet ventilation for Nd-YAG laser. *Br J Anaesth* 1990;**65**:749–53.
70 Hovagim AR, Vitkun SA, Manecke GR, Reiner R. Arterial oxygen saturation in adult dental patients receiving conscious sedation. *J Oral Maxillofac Surg* 1989;**47**:936–9.
71 Tucker MR, Ochs MW, White RP. Arterial blood gas levels after midazolam or diazepam administered with or without fentanyl as an intravenous sedative for outpatient surgical procedures. *J Oral Maxillofac Surg* 1986;**44**:688–92.
72 Bone ME, Galler D, Flynn PJ. Arterial oxygen saturation during general anaesthesia for paediatric dental extractions. *Anaesthesia* 1987;**42**:879–82.
73 Clapham MCC, Mackie AM. Pulse oximetry: an assessment in anaesthetised dental patients. *Anaesthesia* 1986;**41**:1036–8.
74 Beeby C, Thurlow AC. Pulse oximetry during general anaesthesia for dental extractions. *Br Dent J* 1986;**160**:123–5.

75 Lanigan CJ. Oxygen desaturation after dental anaesthesia. *Br J Anaesth* 1992;**68**:142–5.
76 Hempenstall PD, de Plater RMH. Oxygen saturation during general anaesthesia and recovery for outpatient oral surgical procedures. *Anaesth Intens Care* 1990;**18**:517–21.
77 Standing Dental Advisory Committee. *General anaesthesia, sedation, and resuscitation in dentistry*. London: The Committee, 1990. (DE Poswillo, chairman).
78 Shapiro CM, Flanigan MJ. ABC of sleep disorders: function of sleep. *BMJ* 1993;**306**:383–5.
79 McGinty DJ, Beahm EK. Neurobiology of sleep in lung biology. In: Saunders NA, Sullivan CE eds. *Health and disease: sleep and breathing*. New York: Marcel Dekker, 1984.
80 West P, Kryger MH. Sleep and respiration: terminology and methodology. Symposium on sleep disorders. *Clin Chest Med* 1985;**6**:691–718.
81 Kagan J, Segal J. Sleep: the other third of our lives. In: *Psychology, an introduction*. 6th edn. Orlando: Harcourt Brace Jovanovitch, 1988:325.
82 Phillipson EA. Control of breathing during sleep. *Am Rev Respir Dis* 1978;**118**:909–30.
83 White DP. Central sleep apnea. *Clin Chest Med* 1985;**6**:623–32.
84 Lavie P. Incidence of sleep apnoea in a presumably healthy working population: a significant relationship with daytime sleepiness. *Sleep* 1983;**6**:312–8.
85 Guilleminault C, Commiskey J. Progressive improvement of apnea index and ventilatory response to CO_2 after tracheostomy in obstructive sleep apnea. *Am Rev Respir Dis* 1982;**126**:14–20.
86 Phillipson EA. Sleep disorders. In: Murray JF, Nadel JA, eds. *Textbook of respiratory medicine*. Philadelphia: WB Saunders, 1988:1841–60.
87 Bradley TD, Phillipson EA. Central sleep apnea. *Clin Chest Med* 1992;**13**:493–505.
88 Shepard JW, Garrison MW, Grither DA, Dolan GF. Relationship of ventricular ectopy to oxyhemoglobin desaturation in patients with obstructive sleep apnea. *Chest* 1985;**88**:335–40.
89 Deedwania P, Swiryn S, Dhingra R, Rosen KM. Nocturnal atrioventricular block as a manifestation of sleep apnea syndrome. *Chest* 1979;**76**:319.
90 Saito T, Yoshikawa T, Sakamoto Y, Tanaka K, Inoue T, Ogawa R. Sleep apnea in patients with acute myocardial infarction. *Crit Care Med* 1991;**19**:938–41.
91 Bradley TD. Right and left ventricular functional impairment and sleep apnea. *Clin Chest Med* 1992;**13**:459–79.
92 Waldhorn RE. Cardiopulmonary consequences of obstructive sleep apnea. In: Fairbanks DNF, Shiro Fujita, Ikematsu T, Simmons FB, eds. *Snoring and obstructive sleep apnea*. New York: Raven Press, 1987.
93 Shepard JW. Hypertension, cardiac arrhythmia, myocardial infarction and stroke in relation to obstructive sleep apnea. Symposium on breathing disorders in sleep. *Clin Chest Med* 1992;**13**:437–8.
94 Hudgel DW. Mechanisms of obstructive sleep apnea. *Chest* 1992;**101**:541–9.
95 Hudgel DW. The role of upper airway anatomy and physiology in obstructive sleep apnea. *Clin Chest Med* 1992;**13**:383–98.

96 Fleetham JA. Upper airway imaging in relation to obstructive sleep apnea. *Clin Chest Med* 1992;**13**:399–416.
97 Rivlin J, Hoffstein V, Kalbfleisch J, McNicholas W, Zamel N, Bran AC. Upper airway morphology in patients with idiopathic obstructive sleep apnea. *Am Rev Respir Dis* 1989;**129**:355–60.
98 Haponic EF, Smith PI, Bohiman ME, Allen RP, Goldman SM, Bleecker ER. Computerized tomography in obstructive sleep apnoea. *Am Rev Respir Dis* 1983;**127**:221–6.
99 Cooper BG, Veale D, Griffiths CJ, Gibson GJ. Value of nocturnal oxygen saturation as a screening test for sleep apnoea. *Thorax* 1991;**46**:586–8.
100 Ryan PJ, Hilton MF, Boldy DA *et al*. Validation of British Thoracic Society guidelines for the diagnosis of the sleep apnoea/hypopnoea syndrome: can polysomnography be avoided? *Thorax* 1995;**50**:972–5.
101 Mohsenin V, Guffanti EE, Hilbert J, Ferranti R. Daytime oxygen saturation does not predict nocturnal oxygen desaturation in patients with chronic obstructive pulmonary disease. *Arch Phys Med Rehab* 1994;**75**:285–9.
102 Postic WP, Marsh RR. Snoring and obstructive sleep apnea in children. In: Fairbanks DNF, Shiro Fujita, Ikematsu T, Simmons FB, eds. *Snoring and obstructive sleep apnea*. New York: Raven Press, 1987.
103 Eliaschar I, Lavie P, Halpern E, Gordon C, Alroy G. Sleep apneic episodes as indications for adenotonsillectomy. *Arch Otolaryngol Head Neck Surg* 1980;**106**:492–6.
104 Stradling JR, Thomas G, Warley ARH, Williams P, Freeland A. The effect of adenotonsillectomy on nocturnal hypoxaemia, sleep disturbance and symptoms in snoring children. *Lancet* 1990;**335**:249–53.
105 Douglas NJ. Nocturnal hypoxaemia in patients with chronic obstructive pulmonary disease. *Clin Chest Med* 1992;**13**:523–32.
106 Douglas NJ, Asthma at night. *Clin Chest Med* 1985;**6**:663–74.
107 Catterall JR, Douglas NJ, Calverley PM. Irregular breathing and hypoxaemia during sleep in chronic stable asthma. *Lancet* 1982;**i**:301–4.
108 Smith TH, Hudgel DW. Arterial oxygen desaturation during sleep in children with asthma and its relation to airway obstruction and ventilatory drive. *Pediatrics* 1980;**66**:746–51.
109 Mendleson Y, Kent JC. Variations in optical absorption spectra of adult and fetal haemoglobins and its effect on pulse oximetry. *IEEE Trans Biomed Eng* 1989;**36**:844–8.
110 Harris AP, Sendak MJ, Donham RT, Thomas M, Duncan D. Absorption characteristics of fetal haemoglobin at wavelengths used in pulse oximetry. *J Clin Monit* 1988;**4**:175–7.
111 Nijland R, Jongsma HW, Nijhuis JG, Oesburg B, Zijlstra WG. Notes on the apparent discordance of pulse oximetry and multi-wavelength hemoglobin photometry. *Acta Anaesthesiol Scand* 1995;**105**:49–52.
112 Foeg-Anderson N, Siggard-Andersen O, Lundsgaard FC, Wimberly PD. Spectrophotometric determination of hemoglobin pigments in neonatal blood. *Clin Chim Acta* 1987;**166**:291–6.
113 Cornelissen PJH, van Woensel CLM, van Oel WC, de Jong PA. Correction factors for hemoglobin derivatives as measured with the IL282 CO-oximeter. *Clin Chem* 1983;**29**:1555.

114 Zijlstra WG, Buursma A, Koek J, Zwart A. reply to Cornelissen *et al. Clin Chem* 1983;**29**:1556.

115 Robertson NCR, ed. *Textbook of neonatology*. London: Churchill-Livingstone, 1986:722–4.

116 Ryan CA, Barrington KJ, Vaughan D, Finer NN. Directly measured arterial oxygen saturation in the newborn infant. *J Paediatr* 1986; **109**:526–9.

117 Bucher H-U, Fanconi S, Baeckert P, Duc G. Hyperoxia in newborn infants: detection by pulse oximetry. *Pediatrics* 1989;**84**:226–30.

118 Wasunna A, Whitelaw AGL. Pulse oximetry in preterm infants. *Arch Dis Child* 1987;**62**:957–71.

119 Deckardt R, Steward DJ. Non-invasive arterial hemoglobin oxygen saturation versus transcutaneous oxygen tension monitoring in the preterm infant. *Crit Care Med* 1984;**12**:935–9.

120 Cochran DP, Shaw NJ. The use of pulse oximetry in the prevention of hyperoxaemia in preterm infants. *Eur J Pediatr* 1995;**154**:222–4.

121 Delivoria-Papadopoulos M, Roncevic N, Oski FA. Postnatal changes in oxygen transport of term, preterm, and sick infants: the role of red cell 2,3-diphosphoglycerate and adult haemoglobin. *Pediatr Res* 1971;**5**: 235–45.

122 Kelleher JF, Ruff RH. The penumbra effect: vasomotion dependent pulse oximeter artefact due to probe malposition. *Anesthesiology* 1989;**71**: 787–91.

123 Wright IMR. A case of skin necrosis related to a pulse oximeter probe. *Br J Intens Care* 1993:394–8.

124 Trevisanuto D, Ferrarese P, Cantarutti F, Zandardo V. Skin lesions caused by oxygen saturation monitor probe: pathogenetic considerations concerning two neonates. *Pediatr Med Chir* 1995;**17**:373–4.

125 Reiterer F, Fox WW. Multichannel polysomnographic recording for evaluation of infant apnea. *Clin Perinatol* 1992;**19**:871–89.

126 Langbaum M, Eyal FG. A practical and reliable method of measuring blood pressure in the neonate by pulse oximetry. *Pediatr* 1994;**125**: 591–5.

10: Limitations and morbidity

The reputation of the technique of pulse oximetry can be maintained only if its limitations are always borne in mind. Currently this is not the situation, and the indicated value of SpO_2 is relied on totally by most users. It has been shown that there is a marked variability in physicians' understanding, not only of the technique of pulse oximetry but also of the oxygen dissociation curve.[1]

The limitations of currently available pulse oximetry technology may be categorised as *safe* or *dangerous*. The safe limitations are those where the device, despite being unable to indicate a value of SpO_2, makes the observer aware that it is not functioning correctly. The dangerous limitations are those where the pulse oximeter seems to be functioning normally but the indicated value of SpO_2 is incorrect, thereby possibly leading to incorrect management of the patient or a false sense of their wellbeing. These limitations may be further categorised as to whether the problem is due to a *technical* or a *physiological* cause (Box).

Limitations of pulse oximetry

	Safe	Dangerous
Technical	Mechanical artefacts	Accuracy
	Electromagnetic interference	Calibration
		Delay
		"Flooding"
		"Penumbra"
Physiological	Pulse dependence	Abnormal haemoglobins
	Volume	Other absorbants
	Rhythm	Delay
		Pulsatile veins
		(Pigmentation)

Some malfunctions fall into more than one category. Those limitations that are considered to be safe are only so if the pulse oximeter has an oscilloscope-type plethysmograph display. The user should be especially aware of some of the early examples of pulse oximeter which, in the face of artefact or fault condition, locked on to the last good value of SpO_2 that they could calculate.

If pulse oximetry is used for physiological research rather than to detect clinical hypoxia then it is necessary to validate individual pulse oximeters under the conditions of the research.[2,3] It must always be remembered that different models of pulse oximeter may vary in their ability to indicate SpO_2 under varying non-ideal conditions. Trivedi et al.[4] compared five different pulse oximeters under varying conditions of hypoperfusion, probe motion, and exposure to ambient light interference. They concluded that there were significant differences in accuracy under non-ideal conditions, with failure rates from approximately 5% to 50% depending upon the oximeter and the source of interference. No single pulse oximeter performed best under all conditions.

Technical limitations

Mechanical artefacts

Malfunction of the pulse oximeter may be caused by mechanical disturbance between the probe and the anatomy of the patient. As the change in absorption of energy due to the cardiac cycle is only 1–2% of the total absorption, very small mechanical disturbances will have an overwhelming effect on the signal. These will be very obvious on the plethysmograph trace. The quality and complexity of the microprocessor software determines how well a particular pulse oximeter is able to extract the plethysmograph signal from mechanical and other physical interference. All pulse oximeters should display "artefact" or "noisy signal" if the interference makes accurate calculation of SpO_2 impossible. Mechanical artefacts are commonly caused by voluntary and involuntary movements by the patient (shivering, tremor, convulsions etc.). The accuracy of pulse oximetry becomes less reliable if used during exercise tolerance tests.[5]

Langton and Hanning[6] measured the effect of mechanical disturbance. They used industrial vibration testing equipment, to which they attached a subject's hand bearing pulse oximeter probes. In some cases the whole subject was attached to the vibrator. Frequencies were chosen to simulate both shivering and the vibration encountered during transport. Vibration interfered with pulse oximeter function. The time taken to detect hypoxaemia was prolonged, in some cases indefinitely. There were also spurious decreases in SpO_2 which often persisted until the vibration ceased. The probes that behaved best under these conditions were those with a soft lining and springs that exerted firm pressure. Good performance was also associated with pulse oximeters using electrocardiographic synchronisation. Performance was poorer with smaller fingers.

The latest generation of pulse oximeters include advanced digital signal processing such as Masimo-SET, which reduces the failure rate with mechanical artefacts. This is described in Chapter 3. Barker and Shah[7] compared two early generation pulse oximeters with a prototype Masimo-SET technology pulse oximeter under the influence of 3 Hz mechanical vibration of the hand with the probes attached. They found that the vibration significantly affected oximeter function, particularly when the sensors were attached during motion, which requires signal acquisition during motion. The error and drop-out rate was significantly better with the Masimo-SET technology.

In the operating theatre, sources of mechanical interference which may be overlooked are the use of a peripheral nerve stimulator or an evoked-potential stimulator. Keidan *et al.*[8] report that falsely low indications of SpO$_2$ may be caused by these devices.

Replacement of existing pulse oximeters by the latest generation may prove too expensive in the short term. A half-way solution may be a computer algorithm called the Edentec Motion Annotation System, which compares an ECG signal with the pulse signal of existing pulse oximeters.[9]

The problem of mechanical artefacts seems much greater with reflection pulse oximetry.[10] This is because of difficulties in securing the probe, usually to the patient's head. The tighter the probe is fixed, the lower the pulsatile blood flow in the skin immediately under it. The signal may be further degenerated by any oedema under the probe.

Electromagnetic interference

Electromagnetic interference includes several different sources of interference from the electromagnetic spectrum (Figure 10.1). It may be generated by many sources, mostly manmade, but also results from atmospheric events and cosmic noise: even nuclear explosions produce an enormous electromagnetic pulse. Electromagnetic interference is coupled to a piece of electronic equipment by galvanic, capacitive, inductive or electromagnetic (light) means, or by direct spark (static electricity).[12] In general, the more highly complex and

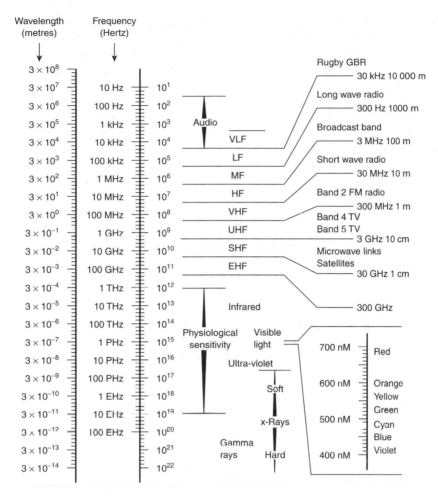

Figure 10.1 Electromagnetic spectrum. Reproduced with permission.[11]

miniaturised a piece of electronic equipment, the more likely it is that it will be susceptible to electromagnetic interference. Pulse oximeters contain much microelectronic circuitry and many microprocessors, and would be very sensitive to electromagnetic interference but for the requirement in their design for a high degree of electromagnetic compatibility – this is now required by statute, especially in equipment on which lives depend.

In pulse oximetry, visible light will interfere with SpO_2 unless the probe is well designed to eliminate its effect. The effects of visible light are far worse if the light source is pulsatile, even if the frequency

143

is as high as 50 or 60 Hz, which is not noticeable to the human eye. Thus problems may occur with fluorescent lighting and poorly designed probes.[13,14] In North America it is common to use xenon arc lighting in operating theatres, and the effect on pulse oximetry is especially severe if this energy is allowed to reach the photodetector.[15] This interference extends into the near infrared wavelengths, and may also include the wavelengths used for infrared diathermy. Infrared heating lamps are also reported to effect the accuracy of pulse oximetry.[16]

The most powerful source of electromagnetic interference that is likely to be encountered is the radiofrequency surgical diathermy unit, which may produce up to 400 W of radiofrequency energy at mixed frequencies. A sign of how well electromagnetic compatibility has been designed into the hardware and software of the pulse oximeter is how well it copes with electromagnetic interference in general, but especially with radiofrequency surgical diathermy.

Dangerous limitations of pulse oximetry

Of the dangerous limitations, calibration and accuracy have already been dealt with in Chapter 4. For completeness, it will only be mentioned in this section that pulse oximeters are calibrated for human adult haemoglobin (HbA) by using fit adults as test subjects. All pulse oximeters become increasingly inaccurate[17,18] when the SaO_2 is < 75%.

The penumbra effect and the errors due to malpositioning of the pulse oximeter probe are a combination of technical and physiological problems. The penumbra effect produces an erroneously low SpO_2 reading when the pulse oximeter probe is malpositioned. This may be due to there being a finite distance between the red and infrared light-emitting diodes, and hence different path lengths for the two wavelengths, especially with babies and children. The penumbra effect has also been noted in adults, which may be due to different path lengths or to pulsatile venules at the tips of the extremities. Kim et al.[19] suggested that the pulsatile venules are a result of the rich arteriovenous anastomoses in the cutaneous circulation at these sites. Cutaneous blood flow may vary from 1 ml/min/100 g of skin to as much as 150 ml/min/100 g in response to thermoregulatory and other vasodilatory stimuli. Cutaneous venules may be pulsatile owing to the arteriovenous anastomoses or the close proximity of pulsatile arterioles. Kelleher and Ruff[20] also speculated that these cutaneous venules might contain desaturated blood from the cutaneous capillaries, and that as the arteriovenous anastomoses render these venules pulsatile, inaccurately low SpO_2 readings are therefore displayed. They also suggested that if the pulse oximeter probe is poorly applied then most of the pulsatile signal is generated by the cutaneous blood flow, with its pulsatile venous component. This would explain why the penumbra effect is less common in conditions causing vasoconstriction, such as hypothermia and peripheral shutdown, when the cutaneous arteriovenous anastomoses are closed, thus reducing the pulsatility of the venules. Inaccurate readings due to the penumbra effect may occur despite a normal appearance of the plethysmograph trace. This is because the trace is generated from one wavelength signal only.

Malpositioning of the pulse oximeter probe was investigated by Barker et al.[21] who found that improperly placed or displaced probes may cause pulse oximeters to become inaccurate. Most pulse oximeters underread, a failsafe condition because it prompts urgent medical attention, but some either overread or failed to follow trends in saturation. These are potentially dangerous situations, as they may induce a false sense of security. Possible explanations include the penumbra effect, and that a weak plethysmograph signal may have a deleterious effect on the ratio of signal to noise and hence its computation.

The most effective ways of guarding against malpositioning and the penumbra effect are good design of the pulse oximeter probe, and also ensuring that the probe is visible to the clinician at all times. Barker et al.[21] also suggested that the observer should maintain a high index of suspicion, especially if there are rapid changes in the SpO_2 value or a discrepancy between the heart rate indicated and the pulse rate. The sensor position should be regularly checked, especially if the patient or the equipment is moved.

Physiological limitations

The pulse oximeter is, by definition, pulse dependent. In many ways this is a vital safety feature, in that an inadequate plethysmograph signal causes complete failure of the device to calculate a value of SpO_2. An abnormal plethysmograph signal causing failure may be classed as safe if it generates an alarm. It would be classed as unsafe if the last value of SpO_2 calculated remained displayed.

The standard pulse oximeter requires a pulse of regular rhythm with the rate and amplitude changing slowly, the AC:DC ratio changing only slightly from beat to beat. The latest generation of pulse oximeters incorporates software that has a greater capability for measuring SpO_2 with irregular heart rhythm and variable pulse amplitude. However, these improvements lead to higher cost.

Falconer and Robinson[22] investigated the effects of reduced pulse pressure on pulse oximetry and found that almost all examples gave similar results as long as the pulse pressure exceeded 20 mmHg. However, significant differences between several pulse oximeters, in both the ability to display readings and the accuracy of reading displayed, occurred when brachial artery occlusion reduced radial artery pulse pressures to 20 mmHg or less.

Because currently available pulse oximeters use only two wavelengths they are unable to distinguish between adult haemoglobin and other normal or abnormal haemoglobins, and will therefore indicate erroneous values of SpO_2. The common dyshaemoglobins, carboxyhaemoglobin and methaemoglobin, are dealt with more fully in Chapter 11.

Other abnormal circulating substances may interfere with two-wavelength pulse oximetry if they absorb energy by significantly different amounts at each wavelength. Bilirubin is often said to interfere with pulse oximetry, but this is untrue.[23] The problem is that pulse oximeters are compared, correctly, with CO-oximeters. However, CO-oximeters operate with wavelengths in the visible part of the spectrum. Bilirubin does affect the calibration of the CO-oximeter, but it does not absorb energy in the range 600–1000 nm, and so does not affect the calibration of pulse oximeters operating in this range. In the presence of severe hyperbilirubinaemia pulse oximetry is more accurate than CO-oximetry.[24]

The physiological dyes (methylene blue, indigo carmine and indocyanine green), when administered intravenously as a bolus, cause inaccuracy in SpO_2 readings.[25] This is because they each absorb energy strongly at 660 nm (Figure 10.2). There have recently been a number of reports of errors in pulse oximetry induced by isosulphan blue, which is often injected intraparenchymally around tumours during surgery[26,27] to map lymphatic drainage. The residual effects of injected dyes may interfere with the accuracy of pulse oximetry for some hours.[28]

Any delays exhibited by a pulse oximeter in indicating a new value of SpO_2 may be dangerous. The delay may be physiological – that is,

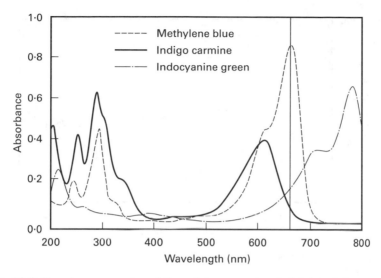

Figure 10.2 Absorbance spectra of three intravenously administered dyes. Dashed line at 660 nm corresponds to one of the wavelengths emitted and sensed by most pulse oximeters. Reproduced with permission.[25]

the time it takes between, say, a reduction in the inspired oxygen concentration and the resultant fall in the oxygen saturation of the haemoglobin passing through the pulse oximeter probe. Many factors may increase this delay, including a decrease in the rate or depth of respiration, or reduced cardiac output. Technical delays are a result of the signal averaging. These delays may increase with low amplitude or irregular pulse.

The most elegant investigation into the response time of pulse oximeters to changes in inspired oxygen concentration was carried out by Young and co-workers[29] at the Royal Air Force Institute of Aviation Medicine. Thirteen pulse oximeters from 10 manufacturers with a total of 26 different probes were used with 11 healthy, non-smoking men. The response times to a 10% step reduction in arterial saturation were measured with an acute decompression technique. Ear probes showed a faster response than finger probes. Two out of the 11 pulse oximeters were significantly slower than the other nine. The response times were also measured for an increase of arterial saturation by suddenly changing the inspired gas, still at an ambient pressure of 380 mmHg, from air to 100% oxygen. Again the ear probes were faster. A summary of results is shown in Figure 10.3. The authors concluded that for the most rapid indication of change in saturation, ear probes should be used.[29]

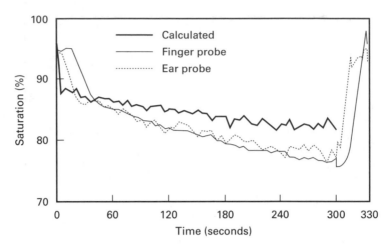

Figure 10.3 Decompression results of Young *et al*. Reproduced with permission.[29]

Pulsatile veins

Pulsatile veins may cause the pulse oximeter to indicate a lower value of SpO_2 than is the true case. Pulsatility in cutaneous venules of the extremities has already been mentioned (the penumbra effect). The pulse oximeter is unable to distinguish between the absorption due to pulsatile veins from that caused by arteries and arterioles. As has been stated already, much of the AC section of the plethysmograph signal may be due to pulsatile cutaneous venules which have an oxygen saturation similar to the arterial saturation, owing to patent arteriovenous communications in the skin. However, if the large venules and veins, which carry haemoglobin with a lower oxygen saturation, are pulsatile then the technique cannot distinguish between artery and vein, and the resulting SpO_2 value will be somewhere between the two. Tricuspid incompetence with regurgitation may cause peripheral veins to become sufficiently pulsatile to render pulse oximetry dangerously inaccurate.[30] Other causes of increased pulsatility in veins include arteriovenous dissociation, right heart block and right atrial myxoma.[31]

Secker and Spiers[32] compared groups of patients with high and low systemic vascular resistance (SVR) in the intensive care unit. SVR was assessed with indwelling pulmonary artery flotation catheters. Patients with low SVR showed a small but significant underestimation of saturation by pulse oximetry. This was hypothesised to be due to the pulse oximeter sensing pulsatile venous flow because of the opening of arteriovenous channels in the skin in septic states.

Pigments

In theory, skin pigmentation should not interfere with the accuracy of pulse oximetry. However, there have been conflicting reports. Gabrielczyk and Buist[33] found no inaccuracies; Cecil et al.[34] suggested that the increased power of light-emitting diodes required to penetrate black skin may be a reason for apparent greater inaccuracy; however, Ries et al.[35] found only a marginal decrease in accuracy but more signal quality problems with highly pigmented subjects. Zeballos and Weisman,[36] comparing CO-oximetry, a Hewlett-Packard eight-wavelength ear oximeter and an early pulse oximeter (Biox IIa) during exercise with black subjects, reported an acceptable accuracy, with the $SaO_2 > 85$ % with the Hewlett-Packard ear oximeter and $SpO_2 > 90$% with the Biox IIa pulse oximeter. They point out that this work needs to be repeated with the newer pulse oximeters.

Peters[37] studied the effect of acrylic artificial nails on pulse oximetry, and found that there was no statistical difference between volunteers with and without false nails which had been applied by a "licensed nail technician"!

Morbidity caused by pulse oximeters

It goes without saying that the use of pulse oximetry in the presence of inflammable gases and vapours and in the vicinity of very high magnetic fields may lead to serious accidents, which are indefensible.

However, there have been several reports of morbidity caused by pulse oximeters. Mechanical pressure has been reported in adults in the critical care situation where the probe has been left in place on the same digit for prolonged periods.[38] Mechanical pressure has also been postulated as the cause of skin necrosis in neonates.[39,40] In these cases pressure was thought to be much more likely as the pathogenetic factor rather than the energy from the LEDs, although this is theoretically possible. In the intensive care situation, digital injury from pulse oximetry may have an incidence as high as 5%, with the highest incidence being in very sick patients with noradrenaline (norepinephrine) infusions reducing the peripheral perfusion.[41]

The Medical Devices Agency, a UK Government-run body, has issued a Safety Notice[42] to all UK hospitals and health care facilities warning that:

- Adhesive tape should not be used to hold pulse oximeter probes in place unless recommended by the manufacturer.
- The site of application should be regularly inspected in accordance with the manufacturer's instructions, or more frequently if indicated by circulatory status and/or skin integrity.
- The site of the probe should be changed every four hours, or more frequently if stated in the manufacturer's instructions.

Photodynamic therapy is increasingly used for the treatment of various cancers. A side effect of this is skin photosensitisation. Cases have been reported of serious digital burns being caused by the use of pulse oximetry during this type of treatment.[43]

Pulse oximeter probe is the formation of a capacitor between the probe circuitry and the living tissues, such that a radiofrequency current could pass during surgical diathermy.

References

1   Stoneham MD, Saville GM, Wilson IH. Knowledge about pulse oximetry among medical and nursing staff. *Lancet* 1994;**344**:1339–42.
2   Wood RJ, Gore CJ, Hahn AG *et al*. Accuracy of two pulse oximeters during maximal cycling exercise. *Aust J Sci Med Sport* 1997;**29**:47–50.
3   Kjuger PS, Longdon PJ. A study of a hospital staffs knowledge of pulse oximetry. *Anaesth Intens Care* 1997;**25**:38–41.
4   Trivedi NS, Ghouri AF, Shah NK, Lai E, Barker SJ. Effects of motion, ambient light, and hypoperfusion on pulse oximeter function. *J Clin Anesth* 1997;**9**:179–83.
5   McGovern JP, Sasse SA, Stansbury DW, Causing LA, Light RW. Comparison of oxygen saturation by pulse oximetry and CO-oximetry during exercise testing in patients with COPD. *Chest* 1996;**109**:1151–5.
6   Langton JA, Hanning CD. Effect of motion artefact on pulse oximeters: evaluation of four instruments and finger probes. *Br J Anaesth* 1990;**65**:564–70.
7   Barker SJ, Shah NK. The effects of motion on the performance of pulse oximeters in volunteers (Revised publication). *Anesthesiology* 1997;**86**:101–8.
8   Keidan I, Sidi A, Gravenstein D. False low pulse oximetry reading associated with concomitant use of a peripheral nerve stimulator and an evoked-potential stimulator. *J Clin Anesth* 1997;**9**:591–6.
9   Poets CF, Stebbens VA. Detection of movement artifact in recorded pulse oximeter saturation. *Eur J Pediatr* 1997;**156**:808–11.

10 Cheng EY, Hopwood MB, Kay J. Forehead pulse oximetry compared with finger pulse oximetry and arterial blood gas measurement. *J Clin Monit* 1987;**4**:223–6.

11 Page-Jones R. *The radio amateur's guide to EMC.* Potters Bar: Radio Society of Great Britain, 1992.

12 Schaffner. *Electromagnetic compatibility, interference suppression and simulation.* Luterbach, Switzerland: Schaffner Elektronik AG, 1985.

13 Hanowell L, Eisele JH Jr, Downs D. Ambient light affects pulse oximeters. *Anesthesiology* 1987;**67**:864–5.

14 Amar D, Neidzwski MS, Wald A, Finck D. Fluorescent light interferes with pulse oximetry. *J Clin Monit* 1989;**5**:135–6.

15 Costarino AT, Davis DA, Keon TP. Falsely normal saturation reading with a pulse oximeter. *Anesthesiology* 1987;**67**:830–1.

16 Brooks TD, Paulus DA, Winkle WE. Infrared heat lamps interfere with pulse oximeters. *Anesthesiology* 1984;**61**:630.

17 Trivedi NS, Ghouri AF, Lai E, Shah NK, Barker SJ. Pulse oximeter performance during desaturation and resaturation: a comparison of seven models. *J Clin Anesth* 1997;**9**:184–8.

18 Carter BG, Carlin JB, Tibballs J, Mead H, Hochmann M, Osbourne A. Accuracy of two pulse oximeters at low arterial hemoglobin-oxygen saturation. *Crit Care Med* 1998;**26**:1128–33.

19 Kim J-M, Arakawa K, Benson KT, Fox DK. Pulse oximetry and circulatory kinetics associated with pulse volume amplitude measured by photoelectric plethysmography. *Anesth Analg* 1986;**65**:1333–9.

20 Kelleher JF, Ruff RH. The "penumbra effect": pulse oximeter artefact due to probe malposition is attenuated by vasoconstriction. *Anesthesiology* 1991;**71**:A372.

21 Barker SJ, Hyatt J, Shah NK, Kao J. The effect of sensor malpositioning on pulse oximeter accuracy during hypoxaemia. *Anesthesiology* 1993;**79**: 248–54.

22 Falconer RJ, Robinson BJ. Comparison of pulse oximeters: accuracy at low arterial pressure in volunteers. *Br J Anaesth* 1990;**65**:552–7.

23 Veyckemans F, Baele P, Guillaume JE, Willems E, Robert A, Clerbaux T. Hyperbilirubinemia does not interfere with hemoglobin saturation as measured by pulse oximetry. *Anesthesiology* 1989;**70**:118–22.

24 Beall SN, Moorthy SS. Jaundice, oximetry and spurious hemoglobin desaturation. *Anesth Analg* 1989;**68**:806–7.

25 Scheller MS, Unger RJ, Kelner MJ. Effects of intravenously administered dyes on pulse oximeter readings. *Anesthesiology* 1986;**65**:550–2.

26 Vokach-Brodsky L, Jeffrey SS, Lemmens HJ, Brock-Utne JG. Isosulfan blue affects pulse oximetry. *Anesthesiology* 2000;**93**:1002–3.

27 Coleman RL, Whitten CW, O'Boyle J, Sidhu B. Unexplained decrease in measured oxygen saturation by pulse oximetry following injection of Lymphazurin 1% (isosulfan blue) during lymphatic mapping procedure. *J Surg Oncol* 1999;**70**:126–9.

28 Chia YY, Liu K, Kao PF, Sun GC, Wang KY. Prolonged interference of patent blue on pulse oximetry readings. *Acta Anaesthesiol Sin* 2001;**39**: 27–32.

29 Young D, Jewkes C, Spittal M, Blogg C, Weissman J, Gradwell D. Response time of pulse oximeters assessed using acute decompression. *Anesth Analg* 1992;**74**:189–95.

30 Stewart KG, Rowbottom SJ. Inaccuracy of pulse oximetry in patients with severe tricuspid regurgitation. *Anaesthesia* 1991;**46**:668–70.

31 Fearnley SJ, Manners JM. Pulse oximetry artefact in a patient with a right atrial myxoma. *Anaesthesia* 1993;**48**:87–8.

32 Secker C, Spiers P. Accuracy of pulse oximetry in patients with low systemic vascular resistance. *Anaesthesia* 1997;**52**:127–30.

33 Gabrielczyk MR, Buist RJ. Pulse oximetry and postoperative hypothermia. *Anaesthesia* 1988;**43**:402–4.

34 Cecil WT, Thorpe KJ, Fibuch EE, Touhy GF. A clinical evaluation of the accuracy of the Nellcor N-100 and the Ohmeda 3700 pulse oximeters. *J Clin Monit* 1988;**4**:31–6.

35 Ries AL, Prewitt LM, Johnson JJ. Skin color and ear oximetry. *Chest* 1989;**96**:287–90.

36 Zeballos RJ, Weisman IM. Reliability of non-invasive oximetry in black subjects during exercise and hypoxia. *Am Rev Respir Dis* 1991;**144**:1240–4.

37 Peters SM. The effect of acrylic nails on the measurement of oxygen saturation as determined by pulse oximetry. *Am Assoc Nurse Anesth J* 1997;**65**:361–3.

38 Richardson NGB, Hale JE. Pulse oximetry – an unusual complication. *Br J Intens Care* 1995;**5**:326–7.

39 Wright IMR. A case of skin necrosis related to a pulse oximeter probe. *Br J Intens Care* 1993;**3**:394–8.

40 Trevisanuto D, Ferrarese P, Cantarutti F, Zandardo V. Skin lesions caused by oxygen saturation monitor probe: pathogenetic considerations concerning two neonates. *Pediatr Med Chir* 1995;**17**:373–4.

41 Wille J, Braams R, van Haren WH, van der Werken C. Pulse oximeter-induced digital injury: frequency rate and possible causative factors. *Crit Care Med* 2000;**28**:3555–7.

42 Medical Devices Agency. Tissue necrosis caused by pulse oximeter probes. MDA SN2001(08) March 2001.

43 Radu A, Zellweger M, Grosjean P, Monnier P. Pulse oximeter as a cause of skin burn during photodynamic therapy. *Endoscopy* 1999;**31**:831–3.

11: Dyshaemoglobins

Abnormal or dyshaemoglobins may have a serious effect on the accuracy of the technique of pulse oximetry. This is because conventional pulse oximeters are calibrated for adult haemoglobin (HbA) and the absorption spectra of adult haemoglobin may differ considerably from those of other forms of haemoglobin.

Carboxyhaemoglobin

Carboxyhaemoglobin has a dangerous effect on conventional two-wavelength pulse oximetry. The pulse oximeter gives a false indication of the patient's wellbeing, as even a very small amount of carboxyhaemoglobin will make the device overread. Figure 11.1 compares the absorption spectrum for carboxyhaemoglobin with those for oxygenated and deoxygenated haemoglobin A. In practice, the displayed SpO_2 is approximately equal to the sum of $SaO_2\%$ + HbCO%.

Different authorities considered the theoretical effect of carboxyhaemoglobin on pulse oximetry differently. Raemer et al.[1] derived their equation from the Beer–Lambert law as:

$$SaO_2 = SpO_2 (1 - 0.932 \, SaCO) + 0.032 \, SaCO$$

Barker and Tremper[2] used the equation:

$$SaO_2 = SpO_2 - 0.9 \, SaCO$$

The manufacturer Nellcor uses the equation:

$$SaO_2 = SpO_2 (1 - SaCO)$$

For practical purposes one may assume that pulse oximeters measure carboxyhaemoglobin, HbCO, as fully oxygenated haemoglobin, HbO_2. This was confirmed in vivo by Vegfors and Lennmarken[3] when they monitored a man who had unsuccessfully attempted suicide by

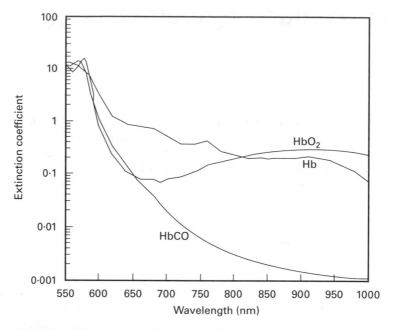

Figure 11.1 Absorption spectra of haemoglobin, oxygenated haemoglobin and carboxyhaemoglobin.

venting the exhaust of his car into the passenger compartment. His oxygen saturation was measured at regular intervals both by pulse oximetry and with a CO-oximeter. The CO-oximeter, which requires discrete blood samples, not only distinguished between oxygenated haemoglobin and carboxyhaemoglobin, but also indicated quantitively the percentages of carboxyhaemoglobin and methaemoglobin. Figure 11.2 shows the change in saturation of haemoglobin as indicated by pulse oximetry and CO-oximetry. During this period the patient was being treated with 50% oxygen in air and recovered without any sequelae. In this case the half-life of carboxyhaemoglobin was approximately 2 hours.

As the conventional pulse oximeter cannot detect the presence of carboxyhaemoglobin, many manufacturers make an allowance in their calibration for a small amount – 1·7% in the case of Ohmeda, based on the statistical average in the fit, healthy, non-smoking population.

Carboxyhaemoglobin is caused by the inhalation of carbon monoxide, which is likely to be present wherever fire is used. It is a colourless, odourless, tasteless, non-irritant gas produced by

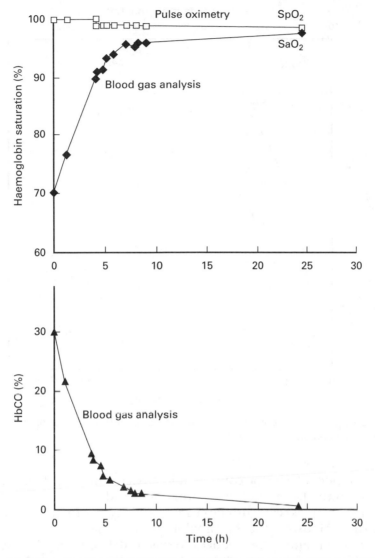

Figure 11.2 Changes in saturation of haemoglobin with oxygen (top) and with carbon monoxide (bottom) during administration of oxygen after a suicide attempt with carbon monoxide. Reproduced with permission.[3]

incomplete combustion of organic material. Carbon monoxide is still a common poison, either deliberately or by accident. Although it is no longer a component of domestic gas, carbon monoxide is a product of partially burnt North Sea gas, as it is of coal. Apart from its effect on haemoglobin, which makes pulse oximetry dangerously inaccurate,

155

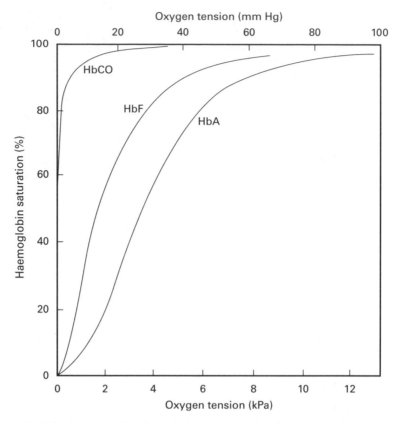

Figure 11.3 Oxyhaemoglobin dissociation curves of carboxyhaemoglobin, fetal haemoglobin and adult haemoglobin.

carbon monoxide has a considerable toxicity unrelated to oxygen delivery to the tissues.[4] Carbon monoxide binds to haem-containing enzymes such as cytochrome P450[5] and cytochrome C. Carbon monoxide binds to the haemoglobin molecule more tenaciously than oxygen and thus reduces oxygen delivery to the tissues. Carboxyhaemoglobin has a bright "cherry red" appearance.

Partial saturation of haemoglobin with carbon monoxide shifts the oxyhaemoglobin dissociation curve of the remaining haemoglobin progressively to the left, and also tends to make the curve less S-shaped and more hyperbolic (the Haldane effect). This leftward shift (Figure 11.3) indicates that the blood *in vivo*, if partially saturated with carbon monoxide, clings to its oxygen with greater tenacity; thus the tissues have much more difficulty in obtaining oxygen from the blood than they do when the oxyhaemoglobin is reduced to a corresponding extent by anaemia.[6]

Causes of carboxyhaemoglobinaemia[9]

Inhalation of carbon monoxide
Tobacco smoking
Fumes from incomplete combustion of carbonaceous material
Coal fumes
Faulty heating systems
Automobiles
Riding in the back of open pick-up trucks
Furnaces
Barbecues/charcoal burners
Fork-lift trucks in enclosed spaces
Fires and conflagrations
Propane-powered machinery

The commonest sources of carbon monoxide are tobacco smoke and the internal combustion engine. Wald *et al.*[7] found that 50% of cigarette smokers had carboxyhaemoglobin concentrations of > 6%, and 5% of > 10%. Concentrations of up to 16% have been recorded in cigarette smokers.[8] Castleden and Cole[9] showed that the carboxyhaemoglobin concentration in an individual smoker is fairly constant and does not normally rise to a maximum at the end of the day. The physiological rate of elimination of carboxyhaemoglobin is proportional to the physical activity of the subject: the greater the activity the faster the elimination. Thus the rate of elimination is much slower overnight than during daytime abstinence from smoking, and a smoker may rise in the morning with a higher carboxyhaemoglobin concentration than a non-smoker.[6] Hence a random estimation of carboxyhaemoglobin will approximate to the mean throughout a 24-hour period. However, giving high concentrations of inspired oxygen will greatly increase the rate of elimination of carboxyhaemoglobin.

Glass *et al.*[10] have formulated a correction formula for SpO_2 related to smoking history.

Passive smoking may be one of the environmental reasons for detectable carboxyhaemoglobin in non-smokers, but the internal combustion engine must also take the blame. A carboxyhaemoglobin concentration of 20% was found in a tobacco-smoking New York taxi driver. Jones *et al.*[11] tested 50 taxi drivers in inner London and found that their carboxyhaemoglobin concentrations ranged between 0·4% and 9·7%, being higher in smokers than non-smokers, and in those on the day shift than those on the night shift, owing to the higher concentration of vehicular traffic. The highest level was found in a smoking night driver.

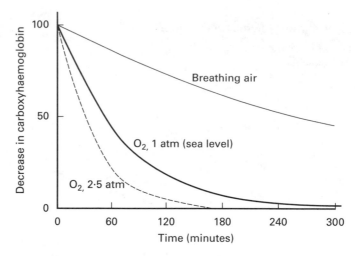

Figure 11.4 Effect of supplemental oxygen on rate of recovery of haemoglobin. Reproduced with permission.[5]

Other important sources of carbon monoxide poisoning are industrial and domestic fires and road traffic accidents. All patients involved in fires have raised carboxyhaemoglobin. Concurrent inhalation of carbon monoxide and cyanide gas is common in both industrial and domestic conflagrations. The cyanide arises from the burning of plastics and polyacrylic fibres.[12] Carbon monoxide and cyanide are synergistic in their effect on the haemoglobin molecule. Carbon monoxide binds to ferrous iron and cyanide to ferric iron.

Patients with carbon monoxide poisoning present with neurological dysfunction, especially a reduced level of consciousness. The cherry-red appearance is rare, late, and much less common than cyanosis.[13] Carbon monoxide poisoning is managed by giving high concentrations of oxygen. Treatment and prognosis have been well reviewed by Gorman and Runciman.[13] Figure 11.4 shows how supplementary oxygen increases the rate of recovery of haemoglobin.

Chronic exposure to low concentrations of carbon monoxide may cause mild or even undetectable symptoms and signs while producing appreciable concentrations of carboxyhaemoglobin, enough to upset greatly the accuracy of the two-wavelength pulse oximeter. Intoxication with carbon monoxide should be treated with high concentrations of inspired oxygen, and many would advocate the use of hyperbaric oxygen.

It cannot be repeated enough that pulse oximeters that overread on all tobacco smokers should arouse a high index of suspicion. Pulse oximeters should never be used with patients who are known to have inhaled carbon monoxide or been involved in any conflagration.

Haemoglobinopathies leading to cyanosis

Cyanosis, a bluish discoloration of the skin and mucous membranes, has been understood since Biblical times to be a sign of disease. Apart from cyanosis due to desaturation of the haemoglobin molecule, it has been recognised for many years that cyanosis may be due to other congenital or acquired defects of the haemoglobin molecule. The commonest dyshaemoglobin causing cyanosis is methaemoglobin. This may be congenital, but is usually acquired. Some very rare congenital haemoglobinopathies may also render patients cyanosed (see below); some of these, designated haemoglobin M, bear some similarities to true methaemoglobin but have slightly different absorption spectra. All of these dyshaemoglobins are associated with a low oxygen affinity and gross inaccuracy of the pulse oximeter. All of the named haemoglobins are rare and hereditary, and their presence is usually easily ascertained by taking a simple history.

Haemoglobins producing cyanosis

M haemoglobins

Hb M_{Osaka}	Hb M_{Boston}	Hb $M_{Hyde\ Park}$
Hb $M_{Saskatoon}$	Hb $M_{Kankakee}$	Hb $M_{Milwaukee}$
Hb M_{Iwate}	Hb $M_{Oldenburg}$	

Other abnormal haemoglobins

Hb_{Torino}	Hb_{Mosbit}	$Hb_{Titusville}$
$Hb_{Raleigh}$	$Hb_{Freiberg}$	Hb_{Moseva}
$Hb_{St\ Louis}$	$Hb_{Louisville}$	$Hb_{Hammersmith}$
Hb_{Chiba}	$Hb_{Okaloosa}$	$Hb_{Seattle}$
$Hb_{Vancouver}$	Hb_{Mobile}	$Hb_{Providence}$
$Hb_{Agenogi}$	$Hb_{Caribbean}$	$Hb_{Beth\ Israel}$
Hb_{Kansas}	Hb_{Burke}	$Hb_{Presbyterian}$
$Hb_{Yoshizuka}$	$Hb_{Peterborough}$	

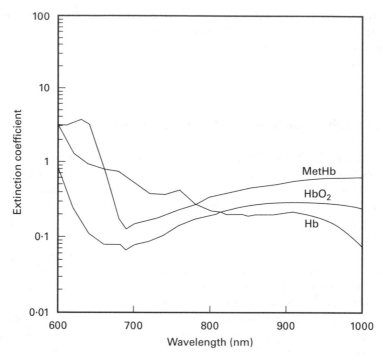

Figure 11.5 Absorption spectra of methaemoglobin, oxygenated haemoglobin and adult haemoglobin.

Acquired methaemoglobinaemia

In this polluted environment in which we now live, the risk of induced methaemoglobinaemia increases year by year. The aetiology may be genetic, idiopathic or toxicological.[14]

Circulating methaemoglobin seriously upsets the calibration of conventional pulse oximeters. Methaemoglobin is haemoglobin with iron oxidised from the normal (or reduced) ferrous (Fe^{2+}) state to the ferric (Fe^{3+}) state. Methaemoglobinaemia refers to greater than the normal physiological concentration of 1–2% methaemoglobin in the erythrocytes. Methaemoglobin is incapable of transporting oxygen. Clinical cyanosis becomes obvious with concentrations greater than 10–15%; spilt blood has an intense "chocolate brown" colour.

Figure 11.5 compares the absorption of methaemoglobin with adult haemoglobin in its oxygenated and deoxygenated states. Pulse oximeters are usually calibrated allowing for 1·5% methaemoglobin, the physiological "normal" level. Any increase above the physiological normal causes the pulse oximeter to indicate a lower oxygen saturation than the true value. The higher the concentration of methaemoglobin, the more the indicated value tends towards 85%. This is because at 85% the absorption ratio between 660 nm and 940 nm is 1:1.

The greatest concern with methaemoglobinaemia is that even if the concentration of methaemoglobin is known or measured before anaesthesia, the concentration may increase during the procedure, so that the calibration of the pulse oximeter alters. Anderson *et al.*[15] reported a case in which benzocaine had been used to anaesthetise the mouth for an awake laryngoscopy and possible intubation. Over the course of the three-hour operation the SpO_2 dropped progressively to the mid-80s, despite an arterial oxygen tension > 200 mmHg. Analysis of the blood with a CO-oximeter showed 26% methaemoglobin.[15]

Causes of methaemoglobinaemia[16]

- Physiological: auto-oxidation by oxygen in formation of oxygen–haemoglobin complexes as part of the physiological function of haemoglobin
- Congenital: haemoglobin M disease, methaemoglobin reductase deficiency
- Acquired methaemoglobinaemia: many chemicals and drugs have been reported to induce methaemoglobinaemia

The Box on p. 162 lists drugs that may produce methaemoglobinaemia.[16,17] Anaesthetists should note the local anaesthetic agents and nitrate and nitrite vasodilators that may cause the level of methaemoglobin to increase during an anaesthetic procedure. Unexpected methaemoglobinaemia may occur as a result of contact with or absorption (orally or transcutaneously) of amyl nitrite, nitrate, or nitrite preservatives in meat; of nitrates in industry; or through contamination of drinking water. A separate Box lists other chemicals that may cause methaemoglobinaemia.[16,18]

Methaemoglobinaemia as a result of exposure to one of these compounds is often referred to as anilism or anilinism, and chemical workers suffering from methaemoglobinaemia may refer to themselves as being "blued up".[18] Table 11.1 shows the symptoms and signs associated with methaemoglobinaemia.

Table 11.1 Symptoms and signs of methaemoglobinaemia.

% Of methaemoglobin	Symptoms or signs
0–15	None
15–20	"Chocolate brown" blood; clinical cyanosis
20–45	Dyspnoea; fatigue; dizziness; lethargy; headache; syncope
45–55	Decreasing level of consciousness
55–70	Coma; convulsions; cardiovascular failure; cardiac arrhythmias
> 70	Death

Drugs producing methaemoglobinaemia

Antimalarials:
   Chloroquine
   Primaquine
   Plasmoquine
Dapsone
Diphenylhydantoin
Ethylenediaminetetra-acetic acid (EDTA)
Glutethimide
Local anaesthetic agents:
   Prilocaine
   Lignocaine
   Benzocaine
Menadione
Methylene blue
Nitrates and nitrites
Para-aminosalicylic acid (PAS)
Phenacetin
Phanazopyridine
Sulphonamides:
   Sulphanilamide
   Sulphapyridine
   Sulphathiazole
Nitroprusside
Nitroglycerine

The management of methaemoglobinaemia can severely affect the operation of the pulse oximeter. General supportive measures are required, including the removal of any further possibility of absorption of any agent leading to methaemoglobinaemia. Asymptomatic patients with methaemoglobin < 20% require close observation for 72 hours after the clearance of the inducing agent. Symptomatic patients require the specific treatment, which is methylene blue (tetramethylthionine chloride) in a dose of 0·1–0.2 ml/kg of a 1% solution (1–2 mg/kg) given intravenously over five minutes. It should

Chemicals causing methaemoglobinaemia

Benzene (industrial solvent)
Nitrobenzenes (oil of Mirbane, dyes,
   explosives, polishes, cheap fragrance)
Aniline (dyestuffs)
Tetranitromethane
Dinitroethyleneglycol
Nitrotoluenes (TNT; explosives)
Dimethylaniline
Tetranitromethylaniline
Para-nitraniline
Ethanolaniline
Para-phenylenediamine
Phenylhydrazine
Acetylphenylhydrazine
Toluidines
Nitrophenols
Paraquat/Diquat
Trional
Chlorates
Potassium chlorate (weedkiller;
   home-made explosives)
Nitrites
Hydroxylamine
Resorcinol

Para-aminophenol
Para-methylaminophenol (Metol,
   photographic developer)
Pyrogallic acid
Antipyrine
Acetanilide
Sulphonal
Cresols (Lysol)
Naphthaline
Copper sulphate
Phenol
Alloxan
Antipyrine
Smoke inhalation
Atsine
Dinitrophenol
Dinitrotoluene

be remembered that large doses of methylene blue may actually induce mild methaemoglobinaemia. Methylene blue has an intense absorption peak at 668 nm which absorbs most of the light at 660 nm; this is interpreted by a pulse oximeter as a reduction in oxygenation.

Methylene blue is also commonly used during diagnostic laparoscopy, when it is injected into the uterus to test the patency of the fallopian tubes.[19] There is often a dip in indicated SpO_2 after methylene blue has been injected through the cervix, as it may be rapidly absorbed into the systemic circulation.

Sickle cell disease and thalassaemia

The conventional two-wavelength pulse oximeter may be used safely with two fairly common types of abnormal haemoglobin, sickle cell disease and thalassaemia, as long as several points are borne in mind.

The sickling disorders result from the inheritance of haemoglobin-S (HbS), either alone or in combination with other abnormal haemoglobins. Haemoglobin-S is caused by a single base mutation in the DNA of adenine to thymine, and this results in the substitution of valine for glutamine at the sixth codon of the β-globin chain. In the homozygous state both genes are abnormal (HbSS), producing sickle cell anaemia; in the heterozygote only one gene is abnormal (HbAS), and this manifests itself as sickle cell trait. As the synthesis of fetal haemoglobin is normal, the disease usually does not manifest itself clinically until fetal haemoglobin decreases to adult levels at about six months of age. The disease is so named because the erythrocytes assume a sickle shape when exposed to hypoxia; they lose their flexibility and are unable to pass so easily through the microcirculation. Sickling may also be precipitated by infection, dehydration, cold or acidosis. Patients feel well unless undergoing a sickling crisis. Those with sickle trait do not suffer a crisis unless the precipitating factors are severe.

The disease or trait occurs mainly in Africans, a quarter of whom carry the gene. It is also found in the Middle East, the Caribbean, the Indian subcontinent and the southern United States.

It is of the utmost importance with sickle haemoglobin that the blood remains sufficiently oxygenated at all times so that sickling does not occur. It is also necessary to understand that there is a shift in the oxyhaemoglobin dissociation curve to the right.

Weston-Smith et al.[20] compared the results of pulse oximetry with those of a blood gas analyser calibrated for HbA. Four patients with sickle cell anaemia (HbSS) with significant desaturation were assessed. Arterial blood samples were taken and injected into the blood gas analyser, which provided results of PaO_2 and SaO_2 based on an algorithm using a P_{50} of 26·85 mmHg, the default value for adult haemoglobin. When blood was withdrawn from the patient the SpO_2 was also measured with a conventional pulse oximeter. An oxyhaemoglobin dissociation curve was also plotted from a sample of blood taken from each patient; a plotting device, as described in Chapter 4, was used. Their results (Table 11.2) show a poor correlation between the pulse oximeter and the arterial oxygen saturation as calculated by the algorithm programmed into the blood gas analyser, but there is a good correlation between pulse oximetry and the saturation calculated by applying the oxygen tension measured by the blood gas analyser to the correct oxyhaemoglobin dissociation curve as measured by the curve plotter.[20] Thus it is safe to rely on the value of oxygen saturation measured by the pulse oximeter in the patient with sickle cell disease or trait. It is, of course, possible to correct the

Table 11.2 Comparison of pulse oximeter and blood gas analyser in sickle cell anaemia[20]

Case No.	Pulse oximeter SpO_2(%)	Blood gas analysis PaO_2 (mmHg)	Blood gas analysis SaO_2 (%)	SaO_2 derived from dissociation curve (%)
1	89	76·1	95·3	88
2	85	74·3	94·5	86
3	76	60·2	92·0	75
4	75	62·0	92·8	76

results of the saturation value circulated by the blood gas analyser by reprogramming into it a value of P_{50} suitable for the blood to be tested, but this would be difficult as the value is not constant between patients with sickle cell anaemia.

Comber and Lopez[21] found that a direct comparison between pulse oximetry and arterial blood gas analysis (ABG) during acute sickle cell crisis showed SpO_2 less than SaO_2 as derived by direct ABG.

Homi et al.[22] showed that low values of SpO_2 are qualitative evidence of hypoxaemia, as they always improved with the administration of high concentration of oxygen. Many stable state homozygous sickle cell patients were persistently mildly desaturated and yet well in themselves. They point out that a *trend* to decreasing SpO_2 was more indicative of deterioration than single values, and therefore frequent recording of SpO_2 in the well state is advantageous.

Fitzgerald and Johnson[23] also confirm that although pulse oximetry slightly underestimates true oxyhaemoglobin saturation, for clinical use it correlates well with CO-oximetry, although in critically ill patients with sickle cell disease if one needs to calculate oxygen content and delivery blood gas sampling is more accurate. This is also confirmed by Kress et al.[24]

The thalassaemias are a group of hereditary haemoglobin abnormalities which, in simple terms, consist of the suppression of the synthesis of adult haemoglobin; there is a compensatory production of fetal haemoglobin, which persists throughout life instead of falling soon after birth. Pulse oximetry indicates the state of saturation of the fetal haemoglobin, but it must be remembered that the oxyhaemoglobin dissociation curve is shifted to the left.

References

1   Raemer DB, Elliott WR, Topulos GP, Philip JH. The theoretical effect of carboxyhaemoglobin on the pulse oximeter. *J Clin Monit* 1989;**5**:246–9.

2   Barker SJ, Tremper KK. The effect of carbon monoxide inhalation on pulse oximetry and cutaneous PO_2. *Anesthesiology* 1987;**66**:677–9.

3   Vegfors M, Lennmarken C. Carboxyhaemoglobinaemia and pulse oximetry. *Br J Anaesth* 1991;**66**:625–6.

4   Haldane JBS. Carbon monoxide as a tissue poison. *Biochem J* 1927;**21**: 1068–75.

5   Vale JA, Meredith TJ. *Poisoning – diagnosis and treatment.* London: Update Books, 1981.

6   Roughton FJW, Darling RC. The effect of carbon monoxide on the oxyhaemoglobin dissociation curve. *Am J Physiol* 1943;**144**:17–31.

7   Wald NJ, Idle M, Boreham J, Bailey A. Carbon monoxide in breath in relation to smoking and carboxyhaemoglobin levels. *Thorax* 1981;**36**: 336–69.

8   Lawtler PJ, Commins BT. Cigarette smoking and exposure to carbon monoxide. *Ann NY Acad Sci* 1970;**174**:135.

9   Castleden CM, Cole PV. Variations in carboxyhaemoglobin levels in smokers. *Br Med J* 1974;**ii**:736–8.

10 Glass KL, Dillard TA, Phillips YY, Torrington KG, Thompson JC. Pulse oximetry correction for smoking exposure. *Military Med* 1996;**161**: 273–6.

11 Jones RD, Commins BT, Cernik AA. Blood lead and carboxyhaemoglobin levels in London taxi drivers. *Lancet* 1972;**ii**:302–3.

12 Gossel TA, Bricker JD. *Principles of clinical toxicology.* London: Raven Press, 1984.

13 Gorman DF, Runciman WB. Carbon monoxide poisoning. *Anaesth Intens Care* 1991;**19**:505–11.

14 Wright RO, Lewander WJ, Woolf AD. Methemoglobinemia: etiology, pharmacology and clinical management. *Ann Emerg Med* 1999;**34**: 646–56.

15 Anderson ST, Hajduczek J, Barker SJ. Benzocaine-induced methemoglobinemia in an adult: accuracy of pulse oximetry with methemoglobinemia. *Anesth Analg* 1988;**67**:1099–101.

16 Hall AH, Kulig KW, Rumack BH. Drug and chemical induced methaemoglobinaemia: clinical features and management. *Med Toxicol* 1986;**1**:253–60.

17 Smith RP, Olson MV. Drug induced methemoglobinemia. *Semin Hematol* 1973;**10**:253–68.

18 Hunter D. *The diseases of occupations*, 6th edn. London: Hodder & Stoughton, 1978.

19 Scott DM, Cooper MG. Spurious pulse oximetry with intrauterine methylene blue injection. *Anaesth Intens Care* 1991;**19**:267–84.

20 Weston-Smith SG, Glass UH, Acharya J, Pearson TC. Pulse oximetry in sickle cell disease. *Clin Lab Haematol* 1989;**11**:185–8.

21 Comber JT, Lopez BL. Evaluation of pulse oximetry in sickle cell anemia patients presenting to the emergency department in acute vasooclusive crisis. *Am J Emerg Med* 1996;**14**:16–18.

22 Homi J, Lvee L, Higgs D, Thomas P, Serjeant G. Pulse oximetry in a cohort study of sickle cell disease. *Clin Lab Haematol* 1997;**19**:17–22.

23 Fitzgerald RK, Johnson A. Pulse oximetry in sickle cell anemia. *Crit Care Med* 2001;**29**:1803–6.

24 Kress JP, Pohlman AS, Hall JB. Determination of haemoglobin saturation in patients with acute sickle chest syndrome: a comparison of arterial blood gases and pulse oximetry. *Chest* 1999;**115**:1316–20.

12: Fetal pulse oximetry

The most recent advance in pulse oximetry is the continuous monitoring of oxygen saturation of the fetus during labour. The earliest form of fetal monitoring was by the intermittent auscultation of the fetal heart sounds using a fetal stethoscope. In the 1960s this was made much easier by the intermittent use of small Doppler ultrasound monitors. Cardiotocography has been routine for the last two decades, involving the *continuous* monitoring of uterine contractions during labour with simultaneous fetal heart monitoring. The fetal heart is monitored either non-invasively by Doppler ultrasound or invasively by the application of a scalp electrode to the fetal head in the normal presentation or to the fetal rump in the breech presentation. Hardcopy recordings of these parameters enable fetal health to be estimated and intervention applied if necessary. It may not be possible to assess fetal distress without taking a capillary sample of fetal blood per vaginam and analysing the blood gases and pH. Unfortunately this technique only gives discrete results, and repeated measurements may be necessary. The advent of the technique of pulse oximetry has led to the development of intrauterine fetal pulse oximetry, which allows continuous real-time monitoring of fetal arterial oxygen saturation and heart rate during labour and delivery.

The special problems related to pulse oximetry *in utero* are listed in the Box.

Problems of *in utero* pulse oximetry

Sensor application sites limited
Reflection mode obligatory
Skin contact necessary
Difficulties with probe attachment
Plethysmograph amplitude smaller (inferior signal-to-noise ratio)
Interference from pulsatility of maternal circulation
Clinician can not observe sensor
Sensor must be waterproof and sterile
$SpO_2 < 70\%$
Calibration difficulties

The design of the probe (Figure 12.1) is significantly different from the conventional probe. As with normal reflection mode probes there

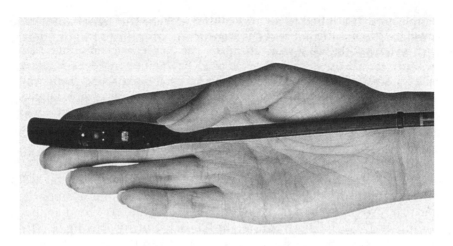

Figure 12.1 Fetal probe.

are two light-emitting diodes (LEDs) and a photodetector, arranged so that the energy reflected back from the tissues is decected by a semiconductor sensor. The wavelengths used in fetal pulse oximetry are different from usual. At the saturation levels below 85% which are normally found with the fetus, the red light energy at 660 nm is absorbed significantly more than at saturations > 85%. Such strongly absorbed energy does not penetrate so deeply into the tissues, and little useful energy is reflected back to the sensor. Therefore, LEDs of 735 nm and 900 nm are used for fetal pulse oximetry.[1] Accurate performance also requires a good overlap in light penetration at the two wavelengths to minimise the effects of tissue homogeneity and a balance in path-length changes arising from perturbations in tissue absorbance.[2] Another theoretical suggestion is the use of three photodetectors at different distances from the LEDs.[3]

Because placement of the probe is difficult and cannot be done under direct vision, there are three electrical contacts associated with the LED–sensor array. These are used to measure the electrical impedance of the fetal skin and to assess probe contact.

The probe is held in position by its careful design and the pressure of the uterine wall. It obviously has to be waterproof to protect its electronic components from amniotic fluid, meconium and blood. It also has to be sterilisable. Faisst et al.[4] improved the application of the probe by applying suction.

The probe's position on the fetus is important for reasons of safety and to obtain a reliable signal. The best position is the cheek or temple area. If applied to an area with dark hair the signal amplitude is reduced; over a caput there is significant shunting of light energy, with a decrease in signal amplitude.

The electronics of the fetal pulse oximeter are significantly more complex than those of the adult version, because the plethysmogram signals are between 2 and 20 times smaller than with adult photoplethysmography. Validation of the signal is therefore more complex. The plethysmogram shape is assessed continuously and compared against a normal expected shape; the validity of the SpO_2 is determined by how close this comparison is. If there is a fetal scalp ECG electrode in place, synchronism of QRS and plethysmograph trace is also used in validating the SpO_2 value. There may be a complete loss of plethysmogram signal during strong uterine contractions, as the pressure on the tissues from the probe eliminates blood flow directly beneath the probe.

Validation

The technique of fetal pulse oximetry has been validated by simultaneous arterial oxygen saturation measurements. This work was done on fetal lambs by Harris et al.[5], who exteriorised the right fetal forelimb to insert a right axillary artery catheter. This was advanced into the left ventricle and then withdrawn 2 cm back into the aortic arch, so that preductal arterial blood samples could be taken. Two fetal pulse oximeter probes were placed over shaved areas of skin. Good correlation between the pulse oximeters and discrete arterial blood samples was shown over the range 6 81% saturation.

Izumi et al.[6] compared fetal saturation $FSpO_2$ during labour with postnatal cord arterial blood samples taken before the first breath, and found good correlation between pulse oximetry and CO-oximetry. They also found that there was a gradual decline in HbF between 37 and 40 weeks of gestation. The HbF concentration at term was between 53% and 88%. This must be taken into account, as although HbF does not affect the calibration of pulse oximetry it does affect CO-oximetry, which uses wavelengths in the visible range of light. This confirms the work of McNamara et al.[7] and Luttkus et al.[8]

Physiological considerations

It would be inappropriate in this text to give a full description of fetal–maternal cardiovascular physiology. Physiology is considered in

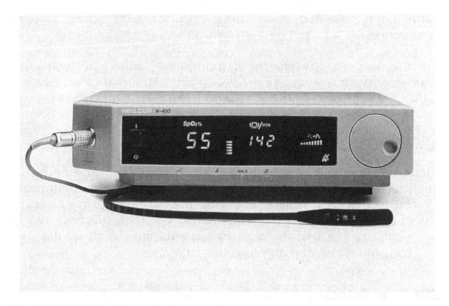

Figure 12.2 Fetal pulse oximeter.

detail by Hanson and Nijhuis,[9] who conclude that the use of FSpO$_2$ is fraught with difficulties in interpretation. Gas exchange between maternal and fetal circulations occurs in the placenta. Despite the relatively low partial pressure of oxygen in the umbilical vein, the fetus is well oxygenated as the oxygen dissociation curve for HbF is shifted to the left of that of HbA (Figure 12.2). Thus, despite the low PO$_2$ this is normally in the range 40–80%.

Fetal pulse oximetry in practice

It is still comparatively early in the history of fetal pulse oximetry for the technique to have gained universal acceptance. More so than pulse oximetry in children and adults, the *trend* of FSpO$_2$ during labour is as important as single values. This is because there is such a wide range of "normal" fetal oxygen saturations.[10] Fetal pulse oximetry does not replace discrete fetal blood sampling at present, as although there is good correlation between FSpO$_2$ and SaO$_2$ from scalp samples, there is poor correlation with fetal scalp blood pH.[11] This has been confirmed by several investigators.[12]

Administration of supplemental oxygen to the mother increases the arterial oxygen saturation in the fetus markedly,[13] the maximum value being attained about nine minutes after administration commences.

There have been few reports of morbidity[14] caused by fetal pulse oximetry so long as the probe was placed atraumatically. Rarely a transient impression of the probe was left on the fetal cheek.[15]

Contraindications to fetal pulse oximetry

Intact membranes have been suggested as a contraindication but, if applied with care, the accuracy of the technique is not compromised by the membranes.[16] Placenta previa obviously presents a serious risk of haemorrhage. Active genital herpes or other infection may be transferred to the fetus by any instrumentation. Intravascular dyes and meconium staining may affect accuracy.

Effect on outcome

Much more work is necessary before fetal pulse oximetry is able to predict the outcome of labour. There is a statistically significant decrease in fetal arterial oxygen saturation during labour in patients with normal and abnormal delivery outcomes.[17] Seelbach-Gobel et al.[18] suggest that $FSpO_2$ below 30% should be the minimum tolerable saturation, as an immediate postpartum pH < 7.2 occurred in more than half the cases in which the saturation was below 30% for more than 10 minutes. They concluded that fetal pulse oximetry did not affect maternal or fetal morbidity. Goffnet et al.,[19] as part of a large multicentre trial, found that there was a significant association between low fetal oxygen saturation ($< 30\%$) and poor neonatal condition. In a review of evidence for a critical theshold of $FSpO_2$, Swedlow[20] concludes that an $FSpO_2$ of 30% represented the third percentile of recorded values of fetal saturation. Statistically this is the dividing line between normal and abnormal fetal saturation.

Saling[21] advises that $FSpO_2$ traces with reduced SpO_2 values, as well as lengthy gaps in the trace, should have urgent scalp blood gas analysis.

References

1   Mannheimer PD, Casciani JR, Fein ME, Nierlich SL. Wavelength selection for low-saturation pulse oximetry. *IEEE Trans Biomed Eng* 1997;**44**:148–58.

2 Mannheimer PD, Fein ME, Casciani JR. Physio-optical considerations in the design of fetal pulse oximetry sensors. *Eur J Obstet Gynecol* 1997;**72(Suppl)**:S9–S19.

3 Graaf R. Tissue optics applied to reflectance pulse oximetry. Groningen, The Netherlands: Thesis, 1993.

4 Faisst K, Kirkinen P, Konig V, Huch A, Huch R. Intrapartum reflectance pulse oximetry: effects of sensor location and fixation duration on oxygen saturation readings. *J Clin Monit* 1997;**13**:299–302.

5 Harris AP, Sendak MJ, Chung DC, Richardson CA. Validation of arterial oxygen saturation measurements in utero using pulse oximetry. *Am J Perinatol* 1993;**10**:250–2.

6 Izumi A, Minakami H, Sato I. Accuracy and utility of a new reflectance pulse oximeter for fetal monitoring during labor. *J Clin Monit* 1997;**13**:103–8.

7 McNamara H, Chung DC, Lilford R. Do fetal pulse oximetry readings at delivery correlate with cord blood oxygenation and acidaemia? *Br J Obstet Gynaecol* 1992;**99**:735–8.

8 Luttkus A, Fengler TW, Friedmann W, Dudenhausen JW. Continuous monitoring of fetal oxygen saturation by pulse oximetry. *Obstet Gynecol* 1995;**85**:183–6.

9 Hanson MA, Nijhuis JG. Pulse oximetry – physiological considerations. *Eur J Obstet Gynecol Reprod Biol* 1997;**(Suppl 1)**:S3–S8.

10 Chua S, Yeong SM, Razvi K, Arulkumaran S. Fetal oxygen saturation during labour. *Br J Obstet Gynaecol* 1997;**104**:1080–3.

11 Johnson N, McNamara H, Montague I, Aumeerally Z, Lilford RJ. Comparing fetal pulse oximetry with scalp pH. *J Reprod Med* 1995;**40**:717–20.

12 East CE, Dunster KR, Colditz PB, Nath CE, Earl JW. Fetal oxygen saturation monitoring in labour: an analysis of 118 cases. *Aust NZ J Obstet Gynaecol* 1997;**37**:397–401.

13 McNamara H, Johnson N, Lilford R. The effect on fetal arteriolar oxygen saturation resulting from giving oxygen to the mother measured by pulse oximetry. *Br J Obstet Gynaecol* 1993;**100**:446–9.

14 Maeselm A, Martensson L, Gudmundsson S, Marsal K. Fetal pulse oximetry. A methodological study. *Acta Obstet Gynecol Scand* 1996;**75**: 144–8.

15 Luttkus AK, Friedmann W, Thomas S, Dimer JA, Dudenhausen JW. The safety of fetal pulse oximetry in parturients requiring fetal scalp blood sampling. *Obstet Gynecol* 1997;**90**:533–7.

16 Elchalal U, Weissman A, Abramov Y, Abramov D, Weinstein D. Intrapartum fetal pulse oximetry: present and future. *Int J Gynecol Obstet* 1995;**50**:131–7.

17 Dildy GA, van den Berg PP, Katz M *et al.* Intrapartum fetal pulse oximetry: oxygen saturation trends during labor and relation to delivery outcome. *Am J Obstet Gynecol* 1994;**171**:679–84.

18 Seelbach-Gohel B, Butterwegge M, Kuhnert M, Heupel M. Fetal reflectance pulse oximetry sub partu. Experiences – prognostic significance and consequences. *Zeitschr Geburtsh Perinatol* 1994;**198**: 67–71.

19 Goffnet F, Langer B, Carbonne B *et al*. Multicenter study on the clinical value of fetal pulse oximetry. I. Methodologic evaluation. The French Study Group on Fetal Pulse Oximetry. *Am J Obstet Gynecol* 1997;**177**: 1238–46.

20 Swedlow DB. *Review of evidence for a fetal SpO$_2$ critical threshold of 30%. Perinatal Reference Note No 2*. Pleasanton, CA: Nellcor Puritan Bennett, 1997.

21 Saling E. Fetal pulse oximetry during labor: issues and recommendations for clinical use. *J Perinatal Med* 1996;**24**:467–78.

Index

Page numbers in **bold** type refer to figures; those in *italic* refer to tables or boxed material.